ANTI-INFLAMMATORY COOKBOOK FOR BEGINNERS 2023 EDITION

1500 Days of Easy and Tasty Recipes to Reduce Inflammation and Improve Your Immune System and Health Through Balanced Nutrition. 28-Day Meal Plan

Stacy Haves

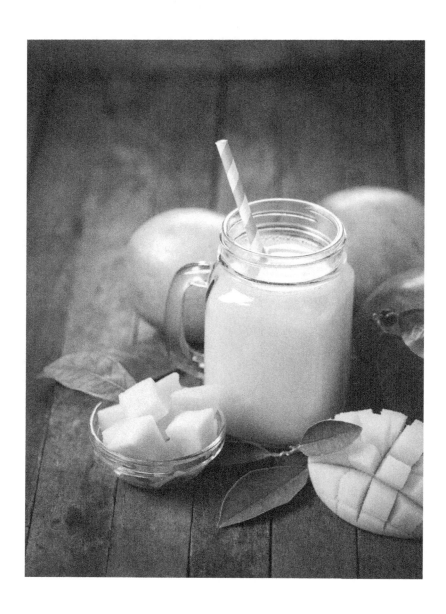

TABLE OF CONTENTS

INTRODUCTION

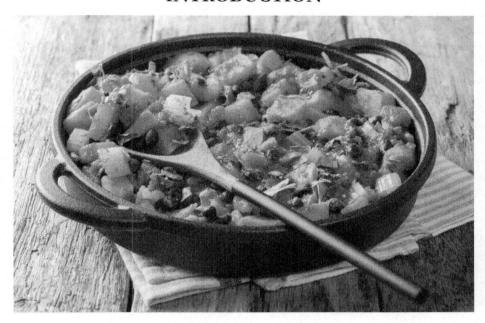

The body's immune system initiates inflammation, a complex biological reaction, in response to injury, infection, or toxins. It is an essential component of the body's natural defense system and aids in removing harmful stimuli and promoting recovery. However, if the inflammation persists long, it can cause various illnesses like cancer, diabetes, heart disease, and inflammatory disorders.

The good news is that research has shown that while some foods can cause inflammation to increase, others can help decrease inflammation in the body. The Anti-Inflammatory Diet, which aims to improve general health and lessen inflammation in the body, was created as a result.

We will examine the foundations of the anti-inflammatory diet in this book and offer helpful advice on how to integrate it into your daily routine. We'll talk about the kinds of foods that can exacerbate inflammation as well as those that can help decrease it. We will also discuss the advantages of eating a diet low in inflammation, such as better gut health, a lower chance of developing chronic illnesses, and more energy.

We will also explore the different forms of inflammation, their signs and symptoms, and treatment options. We will review lifestyle modifications, such as stress reduction, regular exercise, and adequate sleep, that can help reduce inflammation and enhance general health.

This book will give you the information and resources you need to accomplish your goals, whether they are to lessen inflammation, enhance gut health, or live a healthier lifestyle. When you finish reading this book, we hope you will know more about the anti-inflammatory diet and how it can help you reach your health and well-being goals. So let's start the anti-inflammatory diet journey together for improved health and vitality.

CHAPTER 1: ANTI-INFLAMMATORY DIET

The Anti-Inflammatory diet, which has grown in favor recently to lessen chronic inflammation in the body, will be covered in greater detail in this chapter. This chapter will thoroughly explain what inflammation is, the dangers of persistent inflammation, and how an anti-inflammatory diet can help reduce it. The fundamental causes of inflammation in the body and the distinction between acute and chronic inflammation will first be discussed. Acute inflammation is a normal and required reaction to injury or infection, but when it persists for a long time, it can cause many health issues. Chronic inflammation is thought to speed up aging and has been related to diseases like cancer, heart disease, and arthritis. You can recognize the signs and dangers of each form of inflammation by knowing the difference between acute and chronic inflammation.

The advantages of an anti-inflammatory diet, which has been shown to lower inflammation and support general health and wellness, will be covered. The Anti-Inflammatory diet is a method of eating that prioritizes nutrient-dense foods while reducing processed and inflammatory foods. It is not a fad diet. An anti-inflammatory diet has been shown to assist with gut health, lower the risk of chronic diseases, and boost energy levels.

To follow an anti-inflammatory diet, we'll also offer helpful advice on which foods you should consume and which ones you should avoid. Whole, nutrient-dense foods such as fruits and veggies, healthy fats, and whole grains are the mainstays of an anti-inflammatory diet. The various foods that are suggested on this diet, as well as those that should be shunned, are listed in a useful chart that we will provide. You can increase the amount of nutrient-dense foods in your diet while decreasing the amount of processed and packaged foods, refined carbs, and bad fats you consume by adhering to the Anti-Inflammatory diet.

We will discuss the anti-inflammatory diet and behavioral modifications that can reduce inflammation and enhance general health. We'll review the value of managing your stress, getting regular exercise, and getting enough sleep and offer helpful advice for incorporating these routines into your everyday life.

By the conclusion of this chapter, you will be better informed about the Anti-Inflammatory diet and how it can help your body heal by reducing inflammation. With this information, you will be better prepared to decide about your nutrition and way of life and to take action to enhance your general health and well-being.

WHAT IS INFLAMMATION?

The body's immune system naturally responds to pain, infection, or tissue damage with inflammation. The body sends white blood cells to the affected region to help protect and heal it when tissue is harmed, or an infection develops. Inflammation symptoms brought on by this process include redness, warmth, swelling, and pain in the affected region.
An immediate reaction, acute inflammation, usually lasts a few days to a few weeks. It aids the body in warding off infection and mending damaged tissue, and it is an essential step in the recovery process. An example of acute inflammation is a cut or scrape on the epidermis, a sore throat, or an ankle sprain.

On the other hand, chronic inflammation is a long-lasting reaction that can last for weeks, months, or even years. It happens when the immune system is continuously engaged, which causes the body to experience mild inflammation. Numerous health issues, including heart disease, cancer, diabetes, and Alzheimer's disease, have been related to chronic inflammation.
Chronic inflammation can harm the body, whereas acute inflammation is a necessary and advantageous reaction. The signs and symptoms of chronic inflammation, potential causes of inflammation, and potential risks will all be covered in the following part.

WHY INFLAMMATION CAUSES HARM TO THE BODY

Inflammation is a normal and essential reaction when the body is injured or infected. It's a method for the body's immune system to defend itself and encourage recovery. Immune cells and inflammatory molecules are transported to the site of the infection or injury during this process, where they work to eliminate harmed tissues and fend off invasive bacteria. On the other hand, persistent inflammation can harm the body when the immune system is continuously engaged and produces a lot of inflammatory molecules, and chronic inflammation results. Numerous factors, such as exposure to environmental toxins, ongoing worry, a poor diet, and persistent infections, can cause this.

Damage to healthy tissues and organs is one of the primary ways that chronic inflammation can hurt the body. The immune system may unintentionally target healthy tissues when overactive, resulting in damage and inflammation. This can impact the emergence of various health issues, including persistent illnesses like heart disease and diabetes and autoimmune diseases like lupus and rheumatoid arthritis.

Chronic inflammation can also hasten the growth of cancerous cells and damage DNA, which contribute to cancer formation. Encouraging the breakdown of collagen and elastin fibers in the skin and obstructing the body's capacity to regenerate and mend cells can also speed up aging. Allergies, gastrointestinal issues, and skin diseases are just a few of the other health issues that can be brought on by chronic inflammation. Histamines, which can result in allergic responses like hives, itching, and swelling, can be released due to inflammation. To lessen their effects, allergy sufferers frequently take antihistamines.

Additionally, persistent inflammation can obstruct the digestive system's regular operation. Irritable bowel syndrome (IBS), inflammatory bowel disease, and leaky gut syndrome can result from damage to the lining of the digestive system. (IBD). Abdominal pain, bloating, and diarrhea are just a few of the symptoms that these diseases can bring on.

The condition of the epidermis can also be impacted by chronic inflammation. The collagen and elastin strands that give skin its elasticity can be harmed, causing early aging and wrinkles. Additionally, dermatitis, rosacea, and other skin disorders like acne can all be exacerbated by chronic inflammation.

Chronic inflammation can harm the body for several causes, including oxidative stress. A mismatch between free radicals and antioxidants in the body leads to oxidative stress. Free radicals are unstable molecules that can potentially harm DNA and cells, which can result in the onset of chronic illnesses like cancer, heart disease, and Alzheimer's. Free radicals are molecules that can be neutralized by antioxidants, which help to shield the body from their damaging impacts.

In addition to encouraging insulin resistance, chronic inflammation can contribute to type 2 diabetes formation. Chronic inflammation can conflict with insulin's ability to function, making it more challenging for cells to take glucose from the bloodstream.

In general, chronic inflammation can harm the body because it can damage healthy tissues and organs, cause the onset of chronic diseases, and speed up the aging process. By being aware of the dangers of chronic inflammation, we can lessen the body's inflammatory response and advance overall well-being and health.

WHAT TO DO ABOUT INFLAMMATION

Combinations of genetic, environmental, and lifestyle variables frequently lead to chronic inflammation. For instance, eating a diet rich in processed foods, refined sugars, and unhealthy fats can cause inflammation in the body, as can exposure to pollution, toxins, and other external stressors. Chronic inflammation over time can harm and scar tissues and organs, resulting in various health concerns. For instance, persistent blood vessel inflammation can cause plaque to accumulate, raising the chance of heart disease and stroke. In conditions like rheumatoid arthritis, joint inflammation can result in pain, stiffness, swelling, and ultimately irreversible harm. Brain inflammation has been linked to the emergence of neurological conditions like Alzheimer's disease.

An anti-inflammatory diet is a good spot to start if you want to reduce inflammation. This eating plan focuses on whole, nutrient-dense meals rich in antioxidants and other anti-inflammatory substances. Some anti-inflammatory foods are leafy greens, berries, fatty fish like salmon, nuts and seeds, olive oil, and turmeric.

Other lifestyle choices can also aid in reducing inflammation in the body, in addition to dietary adjustments. Regular exercise is known to decrease inflammation because it boosts the creation of anti-inflammatory cytokines and aids in immune system regulation. Inflammation can be reduced, and chronic illnesses can be prevented by getting enough sleep and controlling stress.

While changing one's diet and lifestyle to be anti-inflammatory can help decrease inflammation, in some circumstances, medication may be required to control inflammation and stop further damage to the body. Aspirin and ibuprofen are examples of nonsteroidal anti-inflammatory drugs (NSAIDs) that can help to reduce inflammation and alleviate pain, but they can also have side effects and should only be used under the supervision of a healthcare provider. Overall, supporting optimum health and preventing chronic disease requires reducing inflammation. We can lower inflammation and defend our systems from various illnesses by altering our diet and way of life.

STEPS TO TAKE TO PREVENT INFLAMMATION

- **Eat a low-inflammation diet:** An anti-inflammatory diet emphasizes whole, nutrient-dense foods high in fiber, vitamins, minerals, and polyphenols. These meals provide crucial nutrients that support the immune system and aid in cell repair, which reduces inflammation in the body. Leafy greens, colorful fruits and veggies, fatty fish, nuts and seeds, whole grains, and healthy fats like avocado and olive oil are some foods to include in an anti-inflammatory diet.

- **Include anti-inflammatory foods:** Some foods, such as leafy greens, berries, fatty seafood, nuts, and seeds, as well as spices like turmeric, are known to have anti-inflammatory qualities. Including these items in your diet can lessen inflammation and improve your general health. For instance, adding a portion of berries to your breakfast or including a handful of nuts as a snack can be easy methods to include anti-inflammatory foods in your diet.

- **Avoid pro-inflammatory foods:** On the other hand, some foods, such as processed meats, saturated and trans fats, and refined carbs, can cause inflammation. Limiting these items in your diet will help to lower inflammation and safeguard you from chronic illnesses. Sugary beverages, processed snacks, fried foods, and red meat are some foods to restrict or avoid because they promote inflammation.

- **Keep hydrated:** Water consumption is crucial for general health, which includes reducing inflammation. Water supports healthy cellular function and aids in the removal of pollutants from the body, which can help to lessen inflammation. Aim for 8 cups of water a day minimum, and up to more if you are active or in a warm setting.

- **Regular exercise**: is an effective way to lower inflammation in the body. Your body creates anti-inflammatory cytokines during exercise, which aid in reducing inflammation and fostering healing. Try to exercise for at least 30 minutes, most days of the week, with a moderate effort. Exercises that fall under the category of moderate intensity include swimming, dancing, cycling, and brisk strolling.

- **Reduce tension:** By causing the release of stress hormones, chronic stress can cause inflammation in the body. Practice relaxation methods like deep breathing, meditation, or yoga to manage stress and decrease inflammation. Spending time in nature, participating in pastimes you like, or spending time with loved ones are all examples of additional stress-reducing activities.

- **Sleep well:** Sleep is essential for general health, which includes lowering inflammation. Your body creates cytokines while you sleep, which help to lessen inflammation and encourage healing. Aim for 7-8 hours of sleep each night for optimum wellness. Establish a normal bedtime ritual, abstain from caffeine and alcohol before bed, and create a cozy sleeping environment to encourage better sleep.

- **Keep a healthy weight:** Obesity or being overweight can cause persistent inflammation. You can achieve and keep a healthy weight while lowering inflammation by eating a balanced diet and exercising frequently. Consult a registered dietitian or other healthcare experts for advice if you have trouble reaching a healthy weight.

SYMPTOMS OF INFLAMMATION

The body uses inflammation as a normal and essential mechanism to repair damage and fight infection. However, when inflammation persists for an extended period, it can cause harm and dysfunction in various bodily organs and contribute to the emergence of numerous chronic diseases.

When the body's immune system detects an injury or infection, acute inflammation is a transient reaction that develops. In response, the immune system releases white blood cells like neutrophils and macrophages to the affected region. These cells discharge substances like prostaglandins and cytokines that widen and permeabilize blood arteries. As a result, the affected region receives more blood and immune cells, which causes familiar symptoms of inflammation, such as redness, swelling, warmth, and pain.
On the other hand, chronic inflammation is a protracted reaction that can last for weeks, months, or even years. Poor diet, insufficient exercise, worry, and exposure to toxins in the environment can all cause it. Pro-inflammatory cytokines are released in response to persistent inflammation, which can damage tissue and hasten the onset of numerous chronic illnesses like cancer, diabetes, and heart disease.

Additionally, persistent inflammation can alter the body's immune system, causing an overactive immune reaction that attacks healthy cells and tissues. This may exacerbate autoimmune conditions like lupus and rheumatic arthritis.
In conclusion, inflammation is a normal and essential process that aids wound healing and pathogen defense. But persistent inflammation can harm and impair various bodily functions, promoting the growth of numerous chronic illnesses. We can avoid and treat chronic inflammation by being aware of its causes and effects, which will improve health outcomes.

RISKS OF CHRONIC INFLAMMATION

Numerous health risks are linked to chronic inflammation, which also plays a role in the emergence of many chronic illnesses. The long-term harm that chronic inflammation can do to tissues and organs is one of the primary risks. This may cause tissue death, scarring, and lasting harm to tissues that compromise organ function.

A higher chance of contracting several chronic diseases, including heart disease, cancer, diabetes, and Alzheimer's disease, has also been associated with chronic inflammation. Plaque can build up in the vessels due to inflammation in the body, which can obstruct blood flow and harm the heart muscle. Chronic inflammation in the body can harm cells and cause changes that fuel cancer growth.

The following are some of the most important dangers connected to persistent inflammation:

- Chronic inflammation can damage tissues and cells, which increases the chance of developing chronic illnesses like heart disease, diabetes, cancer, and Alzheimer's disease.

- An immune system weakened: Long-term inflammation can weaken immunity, making it harder for the body to fend off infections and diseases.

- An atmosphere where bacteria and viruses can flourish is created by chronic inflammation, which increases the risk of infections.

- Chronic pain: In diseases like arthritis, inflammatory substances can irritate nerves and cause chronic pain.

- Constipation, diarrhea, and other gastrointestinal issues can all be brought on by chronic inflammation of the digestive system.

- Some evidence supports a connection between chronic inflammation and mental health issues like sadness and anxiety.

- Age spots, wrinkles, and other symptoms of aging can appear more quickly because of chronic inflammation.

It is essential to address chronic inflammation to lower the chance of these complications and enhance general health and well-being. One of the best methods to lessen chronic inflammation and the risks that come with it is to eat an anti-inflammatory diet.

CHAPTER 2: PRINCIPLES OF ANTI-INFLAMMATORY DIET

The anti-inflammatory diet's guiding principles are based on the idea that what we consume can greatly influence how much inflammation is present in our bodies. We can lessen chronic inflammation and advance general health by ingesting foods with anti-inflammatory qualities.

Focusing on whole, nutrient-dense foods high in vitamins, minerals, antioxidants, and anti-inflammatory compounds is a crucial component of the anti-inflammatory diet. Consuming as many fruits and veggies, whole grains, lean protein sources, and healthy fats as possible while limiting processed foods, sugar-sweetened beverages, and trans fats is the way to achieve this.

A balanced consumption of omega-3 and omega-6 fatty acids is a key component of the anti-inflammatory diet. Although both fatty acids are necessary for health, the normal Western diet is frequently high in omega-6s, which can increase inflammation. We can help to regulate our fatty acid ratio and encourage anti-inflammatory effects in the body by increasing our intake of omega-3s (found in fatty fish, flaxseed, and chia seeds) while lowering our intake of omega-6s (found in processed foods and vegetable oils).

The anti-inflammatory diet also stresses the significance of consuming various vibrant fruits and vegetables. Fruits and vegetables of various hues contain a variety of phytochemicals and antioxidants that can fight inflammation and prevent chronic illness. In general, the anti-inflammatory diet's guiding principles emphasize eating a varied, whole-foods-based diet that emphasizes nutrient-dense, anti-inflammatory foods while limiting manufactured and inflammatory foods. These principles can help our body's innate capacity to decrease inflammation and advance optimal health.

WHAT IS AN ANTI-INFLAMMATORY DIET?

A diet that places a focus on nutrients that have been shown to lower inflammation in the body is called an anti-inflammatory diet. The diet is founded on the theory that diabetes, cancer, and heart disease are all caused by chronic inflammation. People may lower their risk of getting these and other chronic illnesses by eating a diet high in anti-inflammatory foods.

The Mediterranean diet, whose advantages for health have been widely studied, is comparable to the anti-inflammatory diet. Many fruits and vegetables, whole grains, lean protein sources such as fish and poultry, and healthy fats such as those in walnuts, seeds, and olive oil are generally included in the diet. Additionally, it promotes the use of spices and herbs, both of which have been found to have anti-inflammatory qualities. The diet also strongly emphasizes avoiding foods like processed foods, refined carbohydrates, and meals rich in saturated and trans fats that can cause inflammation. An anti-inflammatory diet also limits red meat, sugar, and booze.

An anti-inflammatory diet's emphasis on whole, barely processed foods is one of its main tenets. To do this, avoid fried foods and quick food high in unhealthy fats, added sugars, and salt. People are urged to prepare at home with fresh, whole ingredients instead.

Research has shown that following an anti-inflammatory diet can have several health benefits, including reduced risk of heart disease, improved brain function, and lower cancer risk. Additionally, it might aid in reducing the signs and symptoms of some inflammatory diseases and conditions, like inflammatory bowel disease and rheumatoid arthritis. The anti-inflammatory diet is based on several important principles, some of which are as follows:

Consuming various fruits and vegetables: can help reduce inflammation because they are high in antioxidants and phytonutrients. At least 5 to 9 servings of fruits and veggies per day, in various hues and varieties, are advised.

Consuming healthy fats: Anti-inflammatory properties of healthy fats, such as omega-3 fatty acids, are well recognized. They are in olive oil, nuts, seeds, and fatty seafood. It is advised to include these foods in the diet routinely.

Limiting or eliminating processed foods: Processed foods, like fast food, fried foods, and sugary treats, are frequently high in bad fats and extra sugars that can cause inflammation. It is recommended to restrict or keep away from these foods where possible.

Choosing whole grains: Whole grains are full of fiber and other nutrients that can help decrease inflammation. Examples of whole grains include brown rice, quinoa, and whole wheat bread. Whole carbohydrates are advised over refined grains, such as white bread and pasta.

Including lean protein: Lean protein sources can help the body get the necessary amino acids without causing inflammation, such as chicken, turkey, fish, and legumes. It is advised to include these foods in the diet routinely.

In conclusion, the anti-inflammatory diet concentrates on eating foods that have been demonstrated to reduce inflammation while avoiding foods that may promote inflammation. People may be able to lower their chance of developing chronic diseases and enhance their general health and well-being by adhering to this diet.

BENEFITS OF AN ANTI-INFLAMMATORY DIET

1. REDUCES INFLAMMATION: As was already stated, an anti-inflammatory diet can aid in reducing the body's chronic inflammation, which can cause several health issues. Following this diet may help people feel less pain in their joints, have better digestion, and have a reduced chance of developing chronic illnesses like diabetes, heart disease, and some types of cancer.

An anti-inflammatory diet, for instance, may help someone with rheumatoid arthritis feel less pain and inflammation in their joints, like how signs of inflammatory bowel disease may lessen with this eating regimen.

2. ENHANCES HEART HEALTH: Heart-healthy foods like fruits, veggies, whole grains, and lean proteins are abundant in the anti-inflammatory diet. People who adhere to this diet may see their blood pressure drop, their cholesterol levels drop, and their chance of heart disease decrease.

An anti-inflammatory diet, for instance, may help someone with high blood pressure see a drop in their measurements. Similarly, following this eating strategy may help someone whose family has a history of heart disease reduce their risk.

3. WEIGHT REDUCTION is encouraged by the anti-inflammatory diet, which places emphasis on whole, nutrient-dense foods and restricts processed and high-sugar foods. This approach can help individuals feel full and satisfied while consuming fewer calories, contributing to weight loss.

For instance, a person attempting to lose weight may discover that eating an anti-inflammatory diet causes them to feel fuller and more satisfied after meals. Similarly, someone who has battled with binge eating and food cravings might discover that following this eating plan helps them better control these impulses.

4. IMMUNE SYSTEM PERFORMANCE IS IMPROVED by several of the anti-inflammatory diet's foods, which are high in vitamins, minerals, and antioxidants. This diet may help people stay healthier and recuperate more quickly from colds and other illnesses.

For instance, someone susceptible to colds may discover that eating anti-inflammatory foods makes them feel ill less frequently. It is like how eating a diet high in immune-boosting foods may help someone recovering from illness discover that their body can better fight infection.

5. ENHANCES MENTAL HEALTH: According to a recent study, an anti-inflammatory diet may also positively affect mental health. People may experience decreased symptoms of depression, anxiety, and other mental health conditions by eating various nutrient-dense foods.

For instance, a person who battles anxiety might discover that eating anti-inflammatory foods makes them feel calmer and more relaxed. Similarly, someone with depression may experience improvements in mood and energy levels by eating foods that support brain health.

6. BETTER DIGESTIVE HEALTH: Digestive problems like bloating, gas, and diarrhea can be brought on by intestinal inflammation. Improved digestion can result from reducing inflammation in the digestive system with an anti-inflammatory diet and a symphony of symphonies. Yogurt and kefir are foods high in probiotics that can enhance gut health by boosting the population of good microorganisms there.

7. REDUCED CANCER RISK: Chronic inflammation has been associated with a higher risk of breast, lung, and several other kinds of cancer. By reducing inflammatory processes in the body, an anti-inflammatory diet can help reduce the chance of cancer. Foods with anti-inflammatory and anti-cancer qualities include berries, green tea, and cruciferous vegetables. Sulforaphane, a substance in broccoli, has been demonstrated to have anti-cancer and anti-inflammatory effects.

8. IMPROVED SLEEP: Chronic inflammation has been associated with bad sleep, which can result in many health problems. Adopting an anti-inflammatory diet can enhance slumber by lowering body inflammation. Nutrients like tryptophan, magnesium, and melatonin, which have been shown to enhance sleep quality and lower inflammation, are abundant in foods like walnuts, turkey, and kiwis.

ANTI-INFLAMMATORY FOODS CHART

An anti-inflammatory food chart illustrates different foods and their anti-inflammatory characteristics. It can be useful in creating a balanced, healthy diet that encourages general wellness.

The list usually includes foods with anti-inflammatory nutrients like antioxidants, vitamins, and minerals. Here is a description of each item on the list of foods that reduce inflammation:

- **Vegetables:** Vegetables are a crucial component of any healthy diet but play a particularly significant role in anti-inflammatory diets. They are abundant in anti-inflammatory nutrients like fiber, vitamins, minerals, and polyphenols. Leafy greens like spinach, kale, and collard greens and cruciferous veggies like broccoli, Brussels sprouts, and cauliflower are examples of vegetables that reduce inflammation.

- **Fruits:** Fruits are abundant in antioxidants, vitamins, minerals, and fiber, just like veggies are. They can assist in lowering inflammation and enhancing general health. Berries, cherries, oranges, and pineapple are a few anti-inflammatory foods.

- **Whole Grains:** A diet low in inflammatory foods should include whole grains like brown rice, quinoa, and whole wheat bread. They also contain vital nutrients like vitamins, minerals, antioxidants, and a lot of fiber to lower inflammation.

- **Healthy Fats:** Not all fats are made equal, especially healthy fats. Some fats, like those in processed snacks and fried meals, can worsen inflammation. However, healthy fats like those in olive oil, nuts, and fatty seafood like salmon can lessen inflammation. Omega-3 fatty acids, which have anti-inflammatory qualities, are abundant in these fats.

- **Lean Proteins:** While protein is necessary for the body's tissue growth and repair, not all proteins are made equal. Red meat does not reduce inflammation, as well as lean proteins like seafood, poultry, and legumes. This is because they contain more minerals, such as omega-3 fatty acids and antioxidants, and less saturated fat.

- **Herbs and spices:** Adding herbs and spices to your meal can help reduce inflammation and improve the taste. Turmeric, ginger, garlic, and cinnamon are a few herbs and seasonings with anti-inflammatory properties.

- **Beverages:** Water is essential for good health generally and can also help to reduce inflammation. Green tea, which is high in antioxidants, and herbal teas with anti-inflammatory qualities like chamomile are other options for anti-inflammatory drinks.

The anti-inflammatory food chart also stresses the importance of restricting or avoiding processed foods, sweetened beverages, and foods high in saturated and trans fats because they can worsen inflammation.

You can aid in reducing inflammation and enhancing your general health by adhering to the anti-inflammatory food chart and concentrating on foods high in antioxidants, vitamins, minerals, and fiber.

FOODS TO AVOID

Avoiding substances that may cause inflammation is a part of the anti-inflammatory diet. The following items should be avoided while following an anti-inflammatory diet:

- **Foods that have been processed:** Processed foods frequently have high concentrations of sugar, sodium, and bad fats, which can cause the body to become more inflammatory. Fast food, packaged snacks, sugary beverages, and frozen meals are a few examples of processed foods.

- **Refined carbohydrates**: In the body, refined carbohydrates are rapidly converted to sugar, which can lead to blood sugar fluctuations and inflammation. White pasta, bread, and rice are some refined carbs.

- **Sugary foods and beverages:** The body may become inflamed due to consuming foods and beverages with a lot of added sugar, such as candy, soda, and baked products. These sweet foods can raise insulin levels and cause obesity, which increases the chance of chronic inflammation.

- **Trans fats:** Known to increase inflammation, trans fats are frequently found in processed meals. A higher chance of heart disease and other chronic illnesses is also associated with these fats. Fried foods, margarine, and many packaged treats are some foods that could contain trans fats.

- **Lean portions of red meat** can be an excellent source of protein and other nutrients, but they can also be high in saturated fats, which can lead to inflammation in the body. Overeating red meat has been associated with a higher chance of heart disease, stroke, and other long-term health issues.

- **Alcohol:** Alcohol can harm the liver and cause inflammation, resulting in various health issues. While following an anti-inflammatory diet, alcohol intake is advised to be kept to a minimum or avoided entirely.

While on an anti-inflammatory diet, these foods should be avoided; it's equally important to concentrate on eating whole, nutrient-dense foods that are highly anti-inflammatory. Among them are berries, leafy vegetables, fatty seafood, nuts, and seeds. People can decrease inflammation and enhance their general health by emphasizing these foods and avoiding inflammatory foods. Awareness that the anti-inflammatory diet is not a one-size-fits-all strategy and that what functions for one individual may not function for another is crucial. Some individuals might discover that some foods on the avoid list have no impact on their inflammation levels, while others might discover that other foods not on this list have that effect. It's crucial to remember that a healthy lifestyle includes many different components, including an anti-inflammatory diet. In addition to regular exercise and stress control, getting enough sleep is crucial for reducing inflammation and enhancing general health.

CHAPTER 3: BREAKFAST RECIPES

1. Avocado and Egg Toast

Making and Duration Time: 7 minutes **Cooking Duration:** 6 minutes **Number of Portions:** 1

Required Material for this Recipe:
- Toasted whole-grain baguette
- Mash 1/2 mature avocado.
- It's one big egg.
- Add a pinch of crushed red pepper
- Pepper and salt

Step By Step Instructions for Recipe:
1. The bread should be toasted until it reaches the required crispness.
2. Prepare a medium-heated nonstick frying pan while the bread is browning.
3. Scramble the egg in the skillet and boil it until the white is firm but the yellow is still runny.
4. On the buttered bread, spread the pureed avocado and season with pepper flakes, salt, and pepper.
5. Place the finished egg on the bread with avocado. Immediately serve.

Nutritional Analysis: Quantity of Energy in Calories: 284, Quantity of Fat: 19g, Quantity of Carbs: 17g, Quantity of Fiber: 7g, Quantity of Protein: 13g

2. Avocado Toast with Egg and Tomato

Making and Duration Time: 11 minutes **Cooking Duration:** 6 minutes **Number of Portions:** 2

Required Material for this Recipe:
- 2 pieces of toasted whole wheat bread
- Avocado, one, mature, mashed
- 2 eggs
- A single-cut tomato
- Pepper and salt

Step By Step Instructions for Recipe:
1. The bread should be toasted.
2. In a dish, mash the avocado and drizzle it over the top.
3. You can make your eggs any way you like in a nonstick pan.
4. Put the eggs and tomato on the bread with the avocado.
5. Add salt and pepper to taste.
6. Pepper granules if you like things spicy.

Nutritional Analysis: Quantity of Energy in Calories: 355, Quantity of Protein: 17g, Quantity of Fat: 23g, Quantity of Carbs: 23g, Quantity of Fiber: 9g

3. Avocado Toast with Smoked Salmon

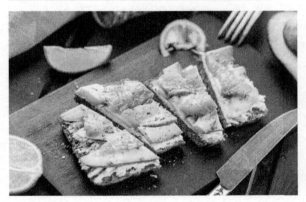

Making and Duration Time: 7 minutes **Cooking Duration:** 5 minutes **Number of Portions:** 1

Required Material for this Recipe:
- Whole-grain bread, one piece
- Avocado, just half part
- Smoked salmon, 2 ounces
- Capers, 1 tablespoon
- The equivalent of one tablespoon of lemon juice
- Pepper and salt

Step By Step Instructions for Recipe:
1. Toast the bread in the oven.
2. Combine the avocado, lemon juice, salt, and pepper in a bowl and mash.
3. Avocados are pureed and spread on bread.
4. Sprinkle some capers and salmon on top.

Nutritional Analysis: Quantity of Energy in Calories: 314, Quantity of Protein: 19g, Quantity of Fat: 19g, Quantity of Carbs: 18g, Quantity of Fiber: 10g.

4. Berry and Almond Butter Smoothie

Making and Duration Time: 6 minutes **Number of Portions:** 1

Required Material for this Recipe:
- Almond milk, 1 cup, sugar-free
- 1/2 cup of a berry mix
- One-half of a mature banana
- Almond butter, 1 teaspoonful
- Add 1/2 tsp. of cinnamon powder
- Vanilla essence, 1/2 tsp (extract)
- 1 tablespoon vanilla protein powder

Step By Step Instructions for Recipe:
1. Combine everything in a blender and blitz until homogeneous.
2. Mix and pour in a tumbler.

Nutritional Analysis: Quantity of Energy in Calories: 290, Quantity of Fat: 15g, Quantity of Carbs: 28g, Quantity of Fiber: 7g, Quantity of Protein: 16g

5. Berry and Chia Seed Pudding

Making and Duration Time: 4 minutes **Cooking Duration:** 2 hours **Number of Portions:** 2

Required Material for this Recipe:
- Almond milk, 1 cup, sugar-free
- 1/4 cup of chia seeds
- Mixed fruit (Berries), half a cup
- 1 Tablespoon of Maple Syrup or Honey (optional)
- 1/2 tsp Vanilla extract

Step By Step Instructions for Recipe:
1. Add vanilla essence and honey or maple syrup to Almond milk and chia seeds.
2. Mix in a handful of assorted fruit.
3. Keep it covered and chilled for at least two hours or overnight.
4. Before serving, mix in some extra milk and stir.

Nutritional Analysis: Quantity of Energy in Calories: 160, Quantity of Fat: 9g, Quantity of Carbs: 16g, Quantity of Protein: 6g, Quantity of Fiber: 10g

6. Berry Chia Pudding

Making and Duration Time: 6 minutes **Chilling Time:** 4 hours **Number of Portions:** 2

Required Material for this Recipe:
- The almond milk for 1
- A quarter cup of chia seeds
- Two teaspoons of honey
- Vanilla essence, 1/2 teaspoon
- 1/2 cup of a berry mix

Step By Step Instructions for Recipe:
1. Combine the chia seeds, almond milk, honey, and vanilla.
2. To avoid clumping, give the combination a few minutes to settle before stirring again.
3. Cool in the fridge for at least four hours, preferably overnight.
4. Top with a variety of fruit and serve.

Nutritional Analysis: Quantity of Energy in Calories: 160, Quantity of Protein: 5g, Quantity of Fat: 9g, Quantity of Carbs: 17g, Quantity of Fiber: 10g

7. Berry Smoothie Bowl

Making and Duration Time: 4 minutes **Number of Portions:** 1

Required Material for this Recipe:
- One serving of chilled berry blend
- Singular Ripe Banana
- Almond milk, half a cup, no sugar added
- 1/4 cup of ground flaxseed
- Honey, one tablespoon's worth

Step By Step Instructions for Recipe:
1. You can make a delicious smoothie by blending together berry fruit, banana, almond milk, chia seeds, and honey.
2. Get a dish and fill it up.
3. Add cereal, cut fruits, and minced almonds.
4. Eat iced.

Nutritional Analysis: Quantity of Energy in Calories: 260 kcal, Quantity of Protein: 6 g, Quantity of Fat: 9 g, Quantity of Carbs: 48 g, Quantity of Fiber: 13 g

8. Blueberry and Almond Butter Smoothie Bowl

Making and Duration Time: 10 minutes **Cooking Duration:** 0 minutes **Number of Portions:** 2

Required Material for this Recipe:
- A single banana, refrigerated
- Frozen blackberries, one cup
- One-half cup of coconut milk
- Almond butter, 2 tablespoons
- 1/4 teaspoon of cinnamon powder
- Extract vanilla, 1/4 teaspoon
- 1/2 cup ground flaxseeds, 1 tablespoon chia seeds, 1 tablespoon of hemp seeds
- 1/tsp grated sugar-free coconut

Step By Step Instructions for Recipe:
1. Process the blueberries, frozen banana, almond butter, cinnamon, and vanilla essence until completely smooth.
2. Split the blended drink between two glasses.
3. Sprinkle with sugar-free shredded coconut, chia and hemp seeds for garnish.

Nutritional information: Quantity of Energy in Calories: 316, Quantity of Protein: 8g, Quantity of Fat: 20g, Quantity of Carbs: 33g, Quantity of Fiber: 9g.

9. Blueberry Almond Chia Seed Pudding

Making and Duration Time: 5 minutes **Chilling Time:** Overnight **Number of Portions:** 2

Required Material for this Recipe:
- Almond milk, 1 cup, sugar-free
- A quarter cup of chia seeds
- Honey: 1 tsp; vanilla extract: 1/4 tsp
- Blueberries, about a quarter cup's worth
- Almonds, chopped, 1/4 cup

Step By Step Instructions for Recipe:
1. Blend chia seeds, honey, vanilla essence, and almond milk together.
2. Thicken it in the fridge overnight by covering it and chilling it.
3. Split the chia seed porridge in half the following morning.
4. Sprinkle strawberries and chopped walnuts on top of each. Serve.

Nutritional Analysis: Quantity of Energy in Calories: 206 kcal, Quantity of Fat: 13 g, Quantity of Carbs: 16 g, Quantity of Fiber: 9 g, Quantity of Protein: 7 g.

10. Blueberry Chia Seed Pudding

Making and Duration Time: 11 minutes **Chilling Time:** 4-6 hours or overnight **Number of Portions:** 2

Required Material for this Recipe:
- Almond milk for 1 cup
- Blueberries, raw, 1/2 cup
- 1/4 cup of chia seeds
- Pure maple syrup measured out to a tablespoon
- Vanilla essence (half a teaspoon), cinnamon powder (one-fourth of a teaspoon)

Step By Step Instructions for Recipe:
1. Blueberries, almond milk, maple syrup, vanilla, and cinnamon should be blended until creamy.
2. The chia seeds and blackberry combination should be thoroughly combined.
3. Put half of the concoction into each of two small containers and chill in the fridge for at least four hours or up to overnight.
4. Serve with extra strawberries on top.

Nutritional Analysis: Quantity of Energy in Calories: 150, Quantity of Protein: 4g, Quantity of Fat: 8g, Quantity of Carbs: 19g, Quantity of Fiber: 9g.

11. Egg White and Spinach Omelet

Making and Duration Time: 6 minutes **Cooking Duration:** 10 minutes **Number of Portions:** 1

Required Material for this Recipe:
- Just 1 cup of young spinach leaves
- Three egg-yolks
- One-fourth cup of tomato slices
- 1/2 cup water, 1 tbsp olive oil
- Pepper and salt

Step By Step Instructions for Recipe:
1. Olive oil should be heated over medium heat in a skillet that won't adhere.

2. Toss the spinach leaves into the pan and cook over medium heat for 1-2 minutes or until wilted.
3. Whisk the yolks of the eggs, salt, and pepper.
4. Bake for 2 to 3 minutes, or until the bottom is firm, after pouring the liquid into the skillet with the spinach.
5. Dice the tomatoes and spread half of them on one surface of the frittata.
6. The egg yolks should be baked for 1-2 minutes. Immediately serve

Nutritional Analysis: Quantity of Energy in Calories: 130, Quantity of Fat: 7g, Quantity of Protein: 13g, Quantity of Carbs: 4g, Quantity of Fiber: 1g.

12. Green Smoothie Bowl with Banana

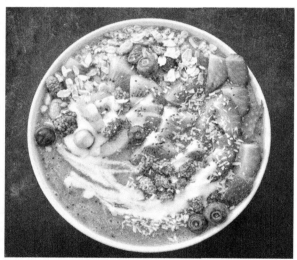

Making and Duration Time: 7 minutes **Number of Portions:** 1

Required Material for this Recipe:
- Almond milk, sweetener-free, 1 cup
- A single cold banana
- Measurement of 1 cup of raw greens
- One-half cup of chilled berry blend
- Just half avocado
- 1/2 cup ground flaxseeds, 1 tablespoon chia seeds
- honey or maple syrup, 1 teaspoon (optional)

Step By Step Instructions for Recipe:
1. Puree a thawed banana, some greens, a few handfuls of assorted fruit, an avocado,

some chia seeds, some honey or maple syrup, and a few shakes of cinnamon.
2. The drink should be served in a dish.
3. Put on whatever you like, whether it's chopped fruit, cereal, or almonds.

Nutritional information: Quantity of Energy in Calories: 360, Quantity of Fat: 21g, Quantity of Carbs: 43g, Quantity of Protein: 8g, Quantity of Fiber: 14g

13. Quinoa and Blueberry Breakfast Bowl

Making and Duration Time: 11 minutes **Cooking Duration:** 20 minutes **Number of Portions:** 2

Required Material for this Recipe:
- One-half cup of ready-to-eat quinoa
- Blueberries, raw, 1/2 cup
- A quarter cup of minced walnuts
- A tablespoon of honey
- 1 gram of cinnamon
- 1/4-liter almond milk

Step By Step Instructions for Recipe:
1. In a small saucepan, mix the prepared quinoa with the almond milk, honey, and cinnamon. Warm the ingredients together over medium heat.
2. Separate the rice into two separate dishes.
3. Fresh strawberries and hazelnuts make a delicious topping. Immediately serve

Nutritional information: Quantity of Energy in Calories: 340, Quantity of Fat: 14g, Quantity of Carbs: 46g, Quantity of Protein: 10g, Quantity of Fiber: 6g.

14. Quinoa Breakfast Bowl

Making and Duration Time: 5 minutes **Cooking Duration:** 25 minutes **Number of Portions:** 2

Required Material for this Recipe:
- Quinoa, 1/2 cup, washed
- Just one water cup
- One-half cup of almond milk
- One-fourth cup of minced walnuts
- Raisins, 1/4 cup
- Ground cinnamon, one teaspoon
- A tablespoon of honey
- 1 banana, cut

Step By Step Instructions for Recipe:
1. Quinoa and water should be combined in a medium saucepan. First, bring to a boil, and then simmer for 20 minutes.
2. Combine the almond milk, walnuts, sultanas, cinnamon, honey, and salt.
3. Continue baking for 5 more minutes, swirling once or twice.
4. Serve in two dishes and garnish with banana slices.
5. Serve.

Nutritional Analysis: Quantity of Energy in Calories: 364, Quantity of Protein: 9g, Quantity of Fat: 10g, Quantity of Carbs: 65g, Quantity of Fiber: 7g

15. Spinach Omelet with Feta

Making and Duration Time: 10 minutes **Cooking Duration:** 10 minutes **Number of Portions:** 2

Required Material for this Recipe:
- Four big Eggs
- 1/4 cup of feta cheese, broken
- Fresh spinach greens, enough for a cup
- Olive oil, 1 tablespoon
- Pepper and salt

Step By Step Instructions for Recipe:
1. Beat the eggs with the seasonings.
2. Olive oil should be heated over medium heat in a skillet that won't adhere.
3. Brown the spinach leaves for a minute or two, or until they wilt, in a skillet.
4. Add the beaten eggs to the spinach and simmer for another 3 to 4 minutes, or until the yolks are firm.
5. Half of the egg should be covered in crumbled feta.
6. Slide the cheese-covered egg onto a platter and fold over the other side.
7. Serve.

Nutritional Analysis: Quantity of Energy in Calories: 235, Quantity of Fat: 18, Quantity of Carbs: 2g, Quantity of Protein: 16g, Quantity of Fiber: 1g

16. Spinach Omelet, Feta, and Dill

Making and Duration Time: 13 minutes **Cooking Duration:** 10 minutes **Number of Portions:** 1

Required Material for this Recipe:
- Two big eggs
- One-fourth cup of raw greens
- 1/4 cup of feta cheese, broken
- Fresh cilantro, minced, 1 tablespoon
- Pepper and salt
- One teaspoon of olive oil

Step By Step Instructions for Recipe:
1. Mix in some salt and pepper to the beaten eggs.
2. Olive oil should be warmed over medium heat in a skillet that won't adhere.
3. Put the spinach in the oven for 1-2 minutes or until it has softened.
4. Bake for 2–3 minutes, or until the eggs are set on the bottom, and then serve over the greens.
5. Sprinkle the feta and parsley over the eggs.
6. Fold the omelet in half with a spoon and heat for another minute or two, until the eggs are set, and the cheddar has dissolved.

Nutritional Analysis: Quantity of Energy in Calories: 272, Quantity of Protein: 19g, Quantity of Fat: 20g, Quantity of Carbs: 3g, Quantity of Fiber: 1g.

17. Spinach Frittata with Mushroom

Making and Duration Time: 10 minutes **Cooking Duration:** 20 minutes **Number of Portions:** 4

Required Material for this Recipe:
- A dozen large yolks
- 1/2 teaspoon of almond extract
- Olive oil, 1 tablespoon
- One-half chopped scallion
- Two chopped garlic cloves
- 1 pound of mushrooms, chopped
- 2 cups raw greens (spinach)
- Pepper and salt

Step By Step Instructions for Recipe:
1. Prepare a 350°F oven.
2. Blend almond milk and yolks together.

3. Olive oil heated over medium heat in a skillet that won't adhere.
4. After a minute or two, add the onion and garlic and continue cooking.
5. Cook for another 2–3 minutes, or until the mushrooms are tender and the spinach is softened, after adding them.
6. Add the egg concoction to the pan with the veggies.
7. If you want crisp borders, cook for another minute or two on the burner.
8. Put in the oven and bake for 10 to 12 minutes, or until the top is firm. Serve.

Nutritional Analysis: Quantity of Energy in Calories: 140, Quantity of Fat: 10g, Quantity of Carbs: 3g, Quantity of Protein: 11g, Quantity of Fiber: 1g

18. Spinach and Mushroom Omelet

Making and Duration Time: 10 minutes **Cooking Duration:** 10 minutes **Number of Portions:** 2

Required Material for this Recipe:
- Four big eggs
- Just 1 tbsp olive oil
- One cup of spinach
- half a cup of chopped mushrooms
- Pepper and salt

Step By Step Instructions for Recipe:
1. Salt and pepper the eggs after they've been beaten.
2. Olive oil should be warmed over medium heat in a skillet that won't adhere.
3. After two minutes of stir-frying the mushrooms, add the greens and cook for another two.
4. After the veggies have been in the oven for five minutes, pour the whisked eggs over them.
5. Bake for another 2 minutes after you've flipped the egg. Keep warm.

Nutritional Analysis: Quantity of Energy in Calories: 214 kcal, Quantity of Protein: 15 g, Quantity of Fat: 17 g, Quantity of Carbs: 3 g, Quantity of Fiber: 1 g.

19. Sweet Potato Breakfast Bowl

Making and Duration Time: 13 minutes **Cooking Duration:** 25 minutes **Number of Portions:** 2

Required Material for this Recipe:
- Scrape and slice one large, sweet potato.
- Olive oil, 1 tablespoon
- A sprinkling of paprika, about 1/2 teaspoon
- Pepper and salt
- 2 servings of raw greens (spinach)
- Two eggs, cooked any way you like
- Avocado, already cut, just 1/4

Step By Step Instructions for Recipe:
1. Turn the oven on to 400 degrees.
2. Combine the sweet potatoes with the oil, spices, salt, and pepper.
3. In order to achieve a delicate and slightly browned sweet potato, spread it out on a plate and roast it for 20-25 minutes.
4. Roasted sweet potato should be divided between two plates.
5. Spinach, chopped avocado, and boiled or cooked eggs make a delicious topping for each dish.

Nutritional Analysis: Quantity of Energy in Calories: 310, Quantity of Fat: 18g, Quantity of Carbs: 22g, Quantity of Protein: 13g, Quantity of Fiber: 7g.

20. Sweet Potato Breakfast Bowl with Cinnamon

Making and Duration Time: 11 minutes **Cooking Duration:** 25 minutes **Number of Portions:** 2

Required Material for this Recipe:
- Remove and slice one large sweet potato.
- Olive oil, 1 tablespoon
- One-half teaspoon of cinnamon powder
- Crushed ginger, 1/2 teaspoon
- one-fourth teaspoon of nutmeg powder
- Pepper and salt
- Two mugs of a salad blend
- A quarter cup of minced walnuts
- Cranberries, dried: 1/4 cups

- Balsamic vinegar, 2 tablespoons

Step By Step Instructions for Recipe:
1. Turn the oven on to 400 degrees.
2. Olive oil, cinnamon, ginger, nutmeg, salt, and pepper should be mixed together and then applied to the sweet potato pieces.
3. To achieve tenderness and a hint of caramelization, roast it for 25 minutes while turning it periodically.
4. In a large dish, toss together the salad leaves, walnuts, and dried cranberries.
5. Sprinkle the balsamic vinegar over the salad leaves and top with the baked sweet potato.

Nutritional Analysis: Quantity of Energy in Calories: 330, Quantity of Protein: 6g, Quantity of Fat: 19g, Quantity of Carbs: 37g, Quantity of Fiber: 8g

21. Sweet Potato and Egg Breakfast Skillet

Making and Duration Time: 11 minutes **Cooking Duration:** 26 minutes **Number of Portions:** 2

Required Material for this Recipe:
- 1 sweet potato, average size, skinned and sliced into cubes
- Half Onion, red
- Diced red capsicum 1
- Two finely minced garlic cloves
- Olive oil, 2 tablespoons
- Four big eggs
- smoky paprika, 1/4 teaspoons
- Pepper and salt
- Garnishing with minced cilantro

Step By Step Instructions for Recipe:

1. Turn the oven on to 400 degrees.
2. Warm the oil in a big skillet over medium heat.
3. Brown the sweet potato for 8-10 minutes, turning periodically, until it is tender.
4. Five minutes into cooking, toss in the minced garlic, chopped red onion, and crushed red pepper.
5. Crack the eggs into the skillet and season with salt, pepper, and smoked paprika.

6. Bake for 8-10 minutes, or until the whites are firm but the yolks are still runny.
7. Finish with a sprinkle of chopped cilantro and serve immediately!

Nutritional Analysis: Quantity of Energy in Calories: 291 kcal, Quantity of Fat: 19 gr, Quantity of Carbs: 20 g, Quantity of Fiber: 4 g, Quantity of Protein: 11 g

22. Sweet Potato-Spinach Frittata

Making and Duration Time: 13 minutes **Cooking Duration:** 20 minutes **Number of Portions:** 4

Required Material for this Recipe:
- 8 large eggs
- 1 sweet potato, average size, skinned and sliced
- 2 cups raw spinach
- Dried thyme, 1/2 teaspoon
- 1/4 teaspoon of onion powder
- Pepper and salt
- One teaspoon of olive oil

Step By Step Instructions for Recipe:
1. Preheat the oven to 375 degrees.
2. Whisk together eggs, thyme, crushed garlic, salt, and pepper.
3. In a large ovenproof pan, boil the olive oil over medium heat. Brown the sweet potato pieces for 5 minutes or until they are soft.
4. Put the spinach in the skillet and cook for a minute or two until it wilts.
5. Add the egg concoction to the skillet with the veggies and stir to combine.
6. Bake for 15 to 20 minutes or until the surface is browned and the eggs are set.
7. Serve by slicing into slices.

Nutritional Analysis: Quantity of Energy in Calories: 224, Quantity of Fat: 14g, Quantity of Carbs: 10g, Quantity of Fiber: 2g, Quantity of Protein: 14g

23. Sweet Potato Hash with Paprika

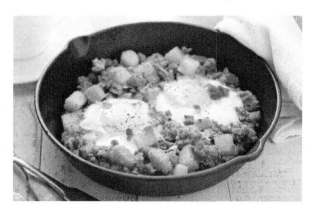

Making and Duration Time: 11 minutes **Cooking Duration:** 21 minutes **Number of Portions:** 2

Required Material for this Recipe:
- Cubed and skinned large, sweet potato.
- 1/2 of a sliced onion.
- Mince up one whole red pepper.
- An olive oil teaspoonful.
- Smoked paprika, 1 tsp.
- Pepper and salt
- 2 eggs

Step By Step Instructions for Recipe:
1. Olive oil, in a skillet, on medium heat.
2. The sweet potato, onion, and pepper should all go into the skillet.
3. Season with salt and pepper and a drizzle of smoky paprika.
4. The sweet potato should be soft and faintly colored after 15 to 20 minutes in the oven, during which time you should turn it periodically.
5. The eggs should be broken over the potato mixture.
6. Cook the eggs to your taste by covering the pan for 3 to 5 minutes.
7. Serve immediately.

Nutritional Analysis: Quantity of Energy in Calories: 308, Quantity of Fat: 14g, Quantity of Carbs: 34g, Quantity of Fiber: 6g, Quantity of Protein: 12g

24. Turmeric and Ginger Oatmeal

Making and Duration Time: 7 minutes **Cooking Duration:** 10 minutes **Number of Portions:** 2
Required Material for this Recipe:
- Roughly one cup of oats
- Almond milk or two glasses of water
- Turmeric powder, one spoonful
- 1 tsp. of ginger powder
- Pepper, about one-fourth teaspoon
- Honey, one tablespoon's worth
- Almonds, pecans, or walnuts, minced (about a quarter cup's worth)

Step By Step Instructions for Recipe:
1. Mix the oats, water/almond milk, spice, ginger, and black pepper.
2. To prepare the oats, bring them to a boil, then reduce heat to medium and stew for 5–7 minutes. Take off the heat and add the honey. Garnish with shredded almonds.

Nutritional Analysis: Quantity of Energy in Calories: 292; Quantity of Fat: 10g; Quantity of Carbs: 46g; Quantity of Protein: 8g; Quantity of Fiber: 7g

25. Turmeric Scramble

Making and Duration Time: 7 minutes **Cooking Duration:** 10 minutes **Number of Portions:** 2
Required Material for this Recipe:
- Four large eggs
- Two teaspoons of butter
- Turmeric, powdered, 1/2 teaspoon
- Ground cumin, 1/2 teaspoon.
- Pepper and salt
- A good amount of spinach
- A single avocado
- One-fourth cup of fresh cilantro, chopped

Step By Step Instructions for Recipe:
1. Olive oil, in a skillet, on medium heat.
2. Add the spices and mix until they release their aroma: turmeric, cumin, salt, and pepper. Scramble the eggs and greens until the eggs are done through.
3. Accompany with fresh cilantro and diced avocado.

Nutritional Analysis: Quantity of Energy in Calories: 320, Quantity of Protein: 17g, Quantity of Fat: 25g, Quantity of Carbs: 9g, Quantity of Fiber: 6g.

CHAPTER 4: LUNCH RECIPES

26. Grilled Salmon and Quinoa Salad

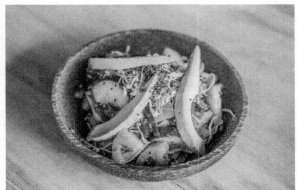

Making and Duration Time: 15 minutes **Cooking Duration:** 17 minutes **Number of Portions:** 2

Required Material for this Recipe:
- Two skinless salmon chunks
- Two-thirds of a cup of rice
- Pepper, scarlet, cut into chunks
- Cucumber, 1/2 slicing
- 1 sliced avocado
- One-fourth cup of chopped red onion
- Olive oil, enough for two teaspoons
- Add the juice of half a lemon, or 2 tbsp.
- One chopped garlic bulb
- Pepper and salt
- Salad, mixed, 2 mugs

Step By Step Instructions for Recipe:
1. Cook the rice as directed and set aside.
2. Prepare a medium fire on the griddle. You can use salt and pepper to season fish pieces. Cook the fish by toasting it for 3–4 minutes per side.
3. Make the dressing by mixing olive oil, lemon juice, garlic, salt, and pepper.
4. Mix rice, vegetables, red bell pepper, cucumber, avocado, and red onion after it has been prepared. Toss in on the sauce to incorporate.

5. Salmon pieces should be served with a rice dish.

Nutritional Analysis: Quantity of Energy in Calories: 490, Quantity of Fat: 32g, Quantity of Carbs: 24g, Quantity of Protein: 28g, Quantity of Fiber: 8g

27. Chicken and Sweet Potato Curry

Making and Duration Time: 17 minutes **Cooking Duration:** 30 minutes **Number of Portions:** 4

Required Material for this Recipe:
- Diced poultry breasts (boneless, skinless) weighing 1 pound
- Two big, skinned, and sliced sweet potatoes.
- Diced scarlet bell pepper, one
- Cubes of 1/2 onion
- Two finely minced garlic cloves
- One Tablespoon of Grated Ginger
- Curry spice, two tbsp
- 1 teaspoon of turmeric powder
- Cayenne pepper, 1/4 tablespoons
- Coconut milk, 1/4 cup
- Olive oil, one tablespoon's worth
- Pepper and salt
- Garnish with fresh parsley

Step By Step Instructions for Recipe:
1. Olive oil should be heated on medium in a big pan.
2. Put in the poultry and roast it on all sides for about 5 to 7 minutes.
3. Fill the skillet with potatoes, bell pepper, onion, garlic, and ginger.
4. Bake for an additional 5 minutes after salting and peppering.
5. Blend the curry, turmeric, and cayenne powder before adding them to the skillet.

6. The poultry and veggies should be almost submerged when you add the water.
7. Simmer for 20–25 minutes or until sweet potatoes are soft.
8. Cook for an additional two to three minutes after adding the coconut milk.
9. Garnish the stew with fresh parsley and serve it steaming.

Nutritional Analysis: Quantity of Energy in Calories: 301, Quantity of Fat: 9g, Quantity of Carbs: 28g, Quantity of Protein: 28g, Quantity of Fiber: 6g.

28. Roasted Chickpea Salad

Making and Duration Time: 17 minutes **Cooking Duration:** 33 minutes **Number of Portions:** 4

Required Material for this Recipe:

- Chickpeas, two cans worth, strained and washed
- Chopped scarlet scallion
  A sliced red and yellow bell pepper
- Two mugs of lettuce
- one-fourth cup of parsley powder
- One-fourth cup of olive oil
- Balsamic vinegar, 2 tablespoons
- Pepper and salt

Step By Step Instructions for Recipe:

1. Preheat the cooking temperature to 375 degrees.
2. Spread the legumes out on a plate and season them with salt and pepper before adding olive oil.
3. Roast legumes for 30 minutes on a grill pan until they are caramelized and crunchy.
4. Combine the roasted legumes, onion, bell pepper, lettuce, and parsley in a bowl.
5. Drizzle with balsamic vinegar and olive oil.
6. Mix until everything is evenly distributed.
7. Serve immediately.

Nutritional Analysis: Quantity of Energy in Calories: 326, Quantity of Fat: 16g, Quantity of Carbs: 33g, Quantity of Fiber: 9g, Quantity of Protein: 11g

29. Grilled Chicken and Vegetable Skewers

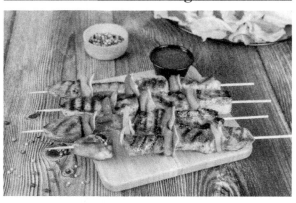

Making and Duration Time: 21 minutes **Cooking Duration:** 15 minutes **Number of Portions:** 4

Required Material for this Recipe:

- Cook four sliced chicken breasts.
- One sliced scarlet onion
- Pepper, red, minced: one, diced
- One cut cucumber.
- a quarter cup of olive oil 1 medium yellow zucchini, diced
- Two chopped garlic cloves
- Dried oregano, one teaspoon
- One and a half thyme leaves, preserved
- Pepper and salt

Step By Step Instructions for Recipe:

1. Get the griddle hot, but not too hot.
2. Skewer the poultry, onions, peppers, cucumber, and zucchini.
3. Olive oil, garlic, oregano, thyme, salt, and pepper should be combined.
4. Apply the olive oil marinade to the skewers.
5. Cook the skewers on the grill for 10 to 15 minutes, flipping them periodically, until the chicken is cooked through, and the veggies are tender.
6. Serve.

Nutritional Analysis: Quantity of Energy in Calories: 345, Quantity of Fat: 19g, Quantity of Carbs: 8g, Quantity of Fiber: 2g, Quantity of Protein: 36g

30. Quinoa Salad with Roasted Veggies

Making and Duration Time: 13 minutes **Cooking Duration:** 27 minutes **Number of Portions:** 4

Required Material for this Recipe:
- Just under a cup of quinoa.
- Water, 2 mugs
- A diced yellow and one red bell pepper
- Thinly sliced red onion, two teaspoons of chopped garlic
- One ounce of olive oil
- Seasonings and spices
- 2 cups of tender spinach, 1/4 ounce of sliced feta cheese

As a seasoning, you can use:
- A quarter of a cup of olive oil
- The equivalent of two tablespoons of balsamic vinegar
- 1 Tbsp. of Honey
- 1 tbsp of Dijon (mustard)
- Spice and seasoning

Step By Step Instructions for Recipe:
1. Turn the oven on to 400 degrees.
2. The quinoa must be washed before being placed in a pot with water. Hold at a boil for a few minutes before reducing heat (to a simmer) for 15–20 minutes, during which time the quinoa should be prepared, and the water consumed.
3. Garlic, olive oil, salt, and pepper should be combined with onion. To broil the veggies until soft and faintly browned, put them on a cookie tray and bake at 400 degrees for 20 to 25 minutes.
4. Mix together the prepared quinoa, vegetables, spinach, and shredded feta.
5. Prepare the dressing by combining the olive oil, balsamic vinegar, honey, mustard, salt, and pepper in a small dish.
6. Toss the quinoa salad with the dressing. You can serve it hot or cold.

Nutritional Analysis: Quantity of Energy in Calories: 346, Quantity of Fat: 21g, Quantity of Carbs: 33g, Quantity of Fiber: 5g, Quantity of Protein: 8g

31. Broiled Salmon with Green Beans and Tomatoes

Making and Duration Time: 13 minutes **Cooking Duration:** 12 minutes **Number of Portions:** 2

Required Material for this Recipe:
- Two fish chunks (salmon)
- Two teaspoons of butter
- Pepper and salt
- Trimmed green beans (about 1/2 pound)
- Tomatoes, cherry: 1 cup
- two sliced bulbs of garlic and two teaspoons of fresh herbs

Step By Step Instructions for Recipe:
1. Turn on the oven to high and foil-line a roasting tray.
2. Season salmon pieces with salt and pepper and drizzle with olive oil. Put them on the sheet pan you have prepared.
3. Toss with the remaining olive oil the green beans, cherry tomatoes, garlic, and parsley, season with salt and pepper to taste.
4. Place the salmon pieces on a baking tray and surround them with the green vegetable concoction.
5. Cook the salmon for 12 minutes and the vegetables for 10 until the fish is opaque and the vegetables are soft and faintly browned. Keep warm.

Nutritional information: Quantity of Energy in Calories: 385, Quantity of Fat: 24g, Quantity of Carbs: 10g, Quantity of Fiber: 4g, Quantity of Protein: 33g

32. Sweet Potato and Chickpea Bowl

Making and Duration Time: 11 minutes **Cooking Duration:** 40 minutes **Number of Portions:** 2

Required Material for this Recipe:
- Two cleaned and sliced medium-sized sweet potatoes
- One drained and washed can of chickpeas
- A teaspoon of each smoky pepper, cumin, and garlic powder
- 1/4 teaspoon of salt
- A Pinch of Pepper

- 2 cups of Kale
- 1 sliced avocado
- Tahini, 2 tablespoons
- The juice of two lemons, measured in tablespoons
- 2 tablespoons of liquid (water)

Step By Step Instructions for Recipe:
1. Turn the oven on to 400 degrees.
2. Combine the legumes, sweet potatoes, smoky paprika, cumin, garlic powder, salt, and pepper.
3. Spread the ingredients out equally on a sheet pan lined with parchment paper. Sweet potatoes usually take about 30–35 minutes to become soft during cooking.
4. Blend together the tahini, lemon juice, and water.
5. The mix should be split between two dishes. Sprinkle the tahini sauce, baked sweet potatoes, legumes, and avocado cubes on top. Serve.

Nutritional Analysis: Quantity of Energy in Calories: 454, Quantity of Fat: 21.8g, Quantity of Carbs: 56.8g, Quantity of Fiber: 15.1g, Quantity of Protein: 14.8g

33. Quinoa and Dark Bean Salad

Making and Duration Time: 15 minutes **Cooking Duration:** 20 minutes **Number of Portions:** 4

Required Material for this Recipe:
- About a cup of quinoa.
- Dark beans from a single can, drained and washed
- Peppers, red, diced
- Half an onion, sliced, and half of the parsley, minced
- Lime Juice, 1/4 Cup
- One-fourth cup of olive oil
- 1/2 tsp. of cumin seed powder
- Use a pinch of salt and a pinch of pepper
- 2 tablespoons of a salad blend

Step By Step Instructions for Recipe:
1. Follow the instructions on the quinoa packaging for baking.
2. Toss together the quinoa, black beans, red pepper, onion, and parsley once they've been prepared.

3. In a dish, mix together the lime juice, olive oil, powdered cumin, salt, and pepper.
4. Toss the quinoa combination with the sauce to cover.
5. Divide the quinoa and black bean combination among four dishes and top with the mixed vegetables. Serve

Nutritional Analysis: Quantity of Energy in Calories: 375 | Quantity of Fat: 16.9g | Quantity of Carbs: 44.4g | Quantity of Fiber: 11.4g | Quantity of Protein: 12.4g

34. Roasted Salmon and Potato Salad

Making and Duration Time: 11 minutes **Cooking Duration:** 25 minutes **Number of Portions:** 2

Required Material for this Recipe:
- Two pieces of fish (salmon)
- 1 large sliced and chopped sweet potato
- Baby greens spinach, two mugs
- One-fourth cup of minced walnuts
- Olive oil, enough for two teaspoons
- Some balsamic vinegar, about a tbsp
- Just 1 tsp honey
- Pepper and salt

Step By Step Instructions for Recipe:
1. Turn the oven on to 400°. Upon a baking tray, spread out some parchment paper.
2. Put the salmon pieces on a roasting pan and season them with salt and pepper.
3. Toss the sweet potato cubes with the olive oil, salt, and pepper in a mixing bowl. Arrange the sweet potato around the salmon pieces on a serving platter.
4. Cook the fish for 20–25 minutes, or until it flakes easily, and soften the sweet potato.
5. In a small dish, combine 1 tablespoon of olive oil with 1 tablespoon each of balsamic vinegar, honey, salt, and pepper.
6. In a separate dish, toss greens with the vinaigrette. Mix.
7. Place the grilled fish and sweet potato on top of the greens and serve. The crushed walnuts should be sprinkled on top.

Nutritional Analysis: Quantity of Energy in Calories: 457kcal, Quantity of Fat: 29g, Quantity of Carbs: 23g, Quantity of Fiber: 4g, Quantity of Protein: 27g

35. Chickpea and Vegetable Sautéed

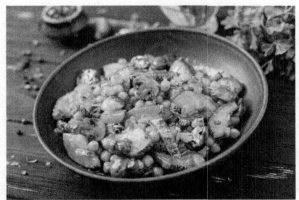

Making and Duration Time: 13 minutes **Cooking Duration:** 17 minutes **Number of Portions:** 2

Required Material for this Recipe:
- Drain and clean 1 can of chickpeas
- 2 cups of a variety of greens (broccoli, bell pepper, mushrooms, carrots, etc.)
- 1 tablespoon olive oil
- Garlic, minced, 1 teaspoon
- 1 tsp of ginger, chopped
- 2 tablespoons of soy sauce
- A tablespoon of honey
- Rice vinegar, 1 tbsp
- Pepper and salt

Dressings on the side:
- scallion chiffonade
- toasted sesame

Step By Step Instructions for Recipe:
1. Oil should be warmed over medium heat in a pan or big pot. Add the medley of veggies and stir-fry for about 7 minutes, or until the veggies are tender.
2. Stir in the garlic and ginger and cook for another minute or two. Stir-fry the legumes for two to three minutes to reheat.
3. Combine the soy sauce, honey, rice vinegar, salt, and pepper in a mixing bowl.
4. Sprinkle the marinade over the veggies and legumes and combine well.
5. Sprinkle the dressing with minced onions and sesame seeds, if preferred, and serve.

Nutritional Analysis: Quantity of Energy in Calories: 335kcal, Quantity of Fat: 10g, Quantity of Carbs: 52g, Quantity of Fiber: 12g, Quantity of Protein: 14g

36. Grilled Salmon Salad

Making and Duration Time: 10 minutes **Cooking Duration:** 10 minutes **Number of Portions:** 2

Required Material for this Recipe:
- A pair of fillets of Salmon
- Four servings of mixed greens
- Sliced avocado, one
- One-third of a cup of sliced cherry tomatoes
- One-fourth cup of chopped red scallion
- Two tablespoons of 100% pure olive oil
- Lemon juice, 2 tablespoons
- 1 chopped garlic bulb
- Pepper and salt

Step By Step Instructions for Recipe:
1. Prepare a medium fire on the griddle.
2. Season the salmon pieces with salt and pepper. Cook the fish on the grill for 5 minutes per side.
3. Olive oil, lemon juice, garlic, salt, and pepper should all be combined to create a sauce.
4. Avocado, cherry tomatoes, and red onion can be added to the greens and blended.
5. Toss the greens with the dressing and pour over the salad.
6. Serve it with a seared salmon piece on each individual dish.

Nutritional Analysis: Quantity of Energy in Calories: 472, Quantity of Protein: 31g, Quantity of Fat: 35g, Quantity of Carbs: 14g, Quantity of Fiber: 8g

37. Roasted Vegetable Quinoa Bowl with Paprika

Making and Duration Time: 13 minutes **Cooking Duration:** 30 minutes **Number of Portions:** 4

Required Material for this Recipe:
- About a cup of quinoa.
- Vegetable stock, two mugs
- One chopped and sliced sweet potato
- Sliced and de-seeded red bell pepper (1)
- Pepper, golden, seeded, and chopped, one

- One courgette cut.
- One medium red scallion cut
- Two tablespoons of 100% pure olive oil
- Dry Oregano, 2 teaspoons
- Smoked paprika, 2 teaspoons
- Pepper and salt
- Parsley, chopped, 1/4 cup

Step By Step Instructions for Recipe:

1. Preheat the oven to 425 degrees.
2. Olive oil, oregano, smoky paprika, salt, and pepper should be used to cover the sweet potato, bell peppers, zucchini, and red onion. Spread the veggies out in a single line on a big baking sheet.
3. To achieve a soft and faintly colored result, grill the veggies for 20–25 minutes, turning periodically.
4. While the veggies are boiling, drain the quinoa in a fine mesh strainer, then add it to the vegetable broth in a medium-sized saucepan.
5. Reduce the heat to medium, cover the skillet, and bring the rice to a boil.
6. Depending on how tender you like your quinoa, it should take about 15–20 minutes to cook in the broth.
7. Divide the quinoa among four plates and fluff it with a spatula.
8. Serve the quinoa topped with sautéed veggies and some fresh parsley.

Nutritional Analysis: Quantity of Energy in Calories: 302, Quantity of Protein: 7g, Quantity of Fat: 9g, Quantity of Carbs: 52g, Quantity of Fiber: 9g

38. Quinoa and Roasted Veggie Salad

Making and Duration Time: 17 minutes **Cooking Duration:** 25 minutes **Number of Portions:** 2-3

Required Material for this Recipe:

- 1 cup of quinoa, washed
- Approximately 2 cups of shredded veggies (e.g., zucchini, bell peppers, eggplant),
- A quarter cup of chopped red scallion
- Add 2 chopped garlic cloves
- Olive oil, enough for two teaspoons
- Oregano, powdered, 1/2 teaspoon
- Basil, desiccated, 1/2 teaspoon

- Pepper and salt
- 1/4 glass of lemon juice
- Parsley, fresh, chopped: 1/4 cup

Step By Step Instructions for Recipe:

1. Preheat the oven to 400°F.
2. Mix the veggies with garlic, oil, herbs, salt, and pepper. Combining ingredients requires a good stir.
3. Roast the vegetables for 20–25 minutes, until they are soft and have acquired a light color, in a single layer on a baking pan.
4. Follow the box directions to cook the quinoa, then set it aside to chill.
5. Put the quinoa, sautéed veggies, red onion, lemon juice, and parsley in a dish and mix well. Serve after a good toss.

Nutritional Analysis: Quantity of Energy in Calories: 292, Quantity of Fat: 12g, Quantity of Carbs: 38g, Quantity of Fiber: 6g, Quantity of Protein: 9g

39. Salmon and Avocado Bowl with Cucumber

Making and Duration Time: 10 minutes **Cooking Duration:** 10 minutes **Number of Portions:** 2

Required Material for this Recipe:

- Two pieces of fish (salmon)
- Pepper and salt
- Avocado, cut, one
- Cherry tomatoes, one cup, divided
- Cucumbers, diced, one cup
- One portion of salad leaves
- Olive oil, 2 tablespoons
- 1/4 glass of lemon juice
- The equivalent of one-fourth teaspoon of garlic powder

Step By Step Instructions for Recipe:

1. Season the salmon with salt and pepper.
2. Olive oil should be warmed over medium heat in a pan. Place the salmon pieces in the pan and roast for four to five minutes on each side.
3. In a small dish, mix the garlic powder, lemon juice, and a pinch of salt.
4. In a separate dish, toss together the mixed greens, cherry tomatoes, and cucumber with the lemon vinaigrette.

5. Separate the salad between two plates and serve each with a piece of grilled salmon and some avocado slices.

Nutritional Analysis: Quantity of Energy in Calories: 482, Quantity of Fat: 36g, Quantity of Carbs: 15g, Quantity of Fiber: 8g, Quantity of Protein: 28g

40. Grilled Chicken Salad with Avocado

Making and Duration Time: 13 minutes **Cooking Duration:** 15 minutes **Number of Portions:** 2

Required Material for this Recipe:
- 2 breasts of poultry, deboned and skinless
- 4 servings of vegetable salad
- Half a cucumber, sliced
- Diced half of an avocado
- Onion, half
- Tomatoes, cherry, 1/2 cup
- The Seeds of a Pumpkin, About a Quarter Cup
- A tablespoon and a half of olive oil
- The juice of half a lemon
- Honey, just a pinch
- Pepper and salt

Step By Step Instructions for Recipe:
1. Prepare a medium fire on the griddle.
2. Season the chicken breasts with salt and pepper.
3. Cook the poultry for 6–8 minutes per side on a hot grill.
4. Dressing can be made by whisking together olive oil, honey, the juice of one lemon, salt, and pepper.
5. Simply combine together the salad leaves, cucumber, avocado, red onion, and cherry tomatoes.
6. The lettuce should be shared between the two dishes.
7. Sprinkle some pumpkin seeds over the salad and top with roasted poultry.
8. Serve the salad by drizzling it with the vinaigrette.

Nutritional Analysis: Quantity of Energy in Calories: 467kcal, Quantity of Fat: 31g, Quantity of Carbs: 18g, Quantity of Fiber: 8g, Quantity of Protein: 34g

41. Mediterranean Quinoa Bowl with Feta

Making and Duration Time: 11 minutes **Cooking Duration:** 23 minutes **Number of Portions:** 2

Required Material for this Recipe:
- One cup of quinoa that has been drained and washed
- Vegetables or low-sodium poultry stock, to the volume of two cups
- Drain and clean half a cup of tinned legumes (chickpeas)
- 1/2 cup of chopped cucumber
- Cut cherry tomatoes to yield 1/2 cup
- Kalamata olives, about a quarter cup, split and sliced
- 2 teaspoons of chopped red scallion
- feta cheese, shredded (about 2 tbsp.
- Parsley, fresh, chopped: 2 teaspoons
- 1 ounce of olive oil
- Lemon juice, 1 teaspoonful
- Dried oregano, 1/2 teaspoon
- Pepper and salt

Step By Step Instructions for Recipe:
1. In a medium pot, bring the broth and quinoa to a simmer.
2. Cover and boil the quinoa for 15–20 minutes, or until soft and the liquid is absorbed, reducing the heat as needed.
3. Olive oil, lemon juice, dried oregano, salt, and pepper should be mixed together to make the sauce.
4. In a large dish, mix the quinoa, cucumber, cherry tomatoes, kalamata olives, red onion, and legumes.
5. Crumble some feta cheese and sprinkle some minced herbs on top of each serving.
6. To serve, drizzle the sauce over the quinoa.

Nutritional Analysis: Quantity of Energy in Calories: 459kcal, Quantity of Fat: 22g, Quantity of Carbs: 52g, Quantity of Fiber: 10g, Quantity of Protein: 16g

42. Grilled Chicken Salad with Balsamic Vinegar

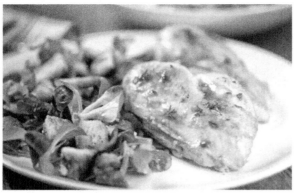

Making and Duration Time: 15 minutes
Cooking Duration: 10 minutes **Number of Portions:** 2

Required Material for this Recipe:
- 2 poultry breasts without bones or flesh
- 4 servings of salad leaves
- One avocado, sliced
- Cherry tomatoes, half a cup
- Cucumber, diced, 1/2 cup
- Thinly cut red onion, about a quarter cup
- Olive oil, enough for two teaspoons
- Balsamic Vinegar, 2 Tablespoons
- Pepper and salt

Step By Step Instructions for Recipe:
1. Prepare a medium fire on the griddle.
2. Season the chicken breasts with salt and pepper.
3. Cook poultry for about 5–6 minutes per side on a grill.
4. Toss together some leaves, avocado, tomatoes, cucumber, and red onion.
5. Olive oil, balsamic vinegar, salt, and black pepper should be mixed together in a dish to make the sauce.
6. The chicken should be cut up and added to the salad.
7. Toss the lettuce with the dressing, then serve.

Nutritional Analysis: Quantity of Energy in Calories: 423, Quantity of Protein: 34g, Quantity of Fat: 29g, Quantity of Carbs: 13g, Quantity of Fiber: 8g

43. Lentil Soup with Paprika

Making and Duration Time: 17 minutes
Cooking Duration: 35 minutes **Number of Portions:** 4

Required Material for this Recipe:
- Red legumes, soaked and washed for a cup
- Two teaspoons of butter
- One diced onion, two minced carrots, and four gallons of veggie stock.
- 2 sliced stems of celery
- 2 garlic bulbs, chopped
- Ground cumin, 1 teaspoon
- Ground cilantro (about 1/2 teaspoon)
- Smoked paprika, 1/2 teaspoon
- Add a pinch of crushed red pepper
- Pepper and salt

Step By Step Instructions for Recipe:
1. Olive oil should be warmed over medium heat in a big pot.
2. All of the vegetables and the garlic and onion should be added. Keep an eye on the vegetables and cook for about 10 minutes, turning periodically.
3. Spice it up with some smoky paprika, cumin, coriander, and crushed red pepper. To add taste while baking, mix continuously for 1 to 2 minutes.
4. To prepare legumes, bring vegetable stock and lentils to a boil, then lower the heat to low and cook for 20–25 minutes. Season with salt and pepper, then serve.

Nutritional Analysis: Quantity of Energy in Calories: 218, Quantity of Protein: 13g, Quantity of Fat: 4g, Quantity of Carbs: 34g, Quantity of Fiber: 14g

44. Grilled Chicken and Veggie Bowls with Quinoa

Making and Duration Time: 15 minutes
Cooking Duration: 10-12 minutes **Number of Portions:** 2

Required Material for this Recipe:
- Two breasts of poultry, skinned and naked
- One scarlet bell pepper, cut
- One golden bell pepper, cut

- One courgette, cut.
- Approximately one tablespoon of olive oil
- A pinch of dried garlic
- Pepper and salt
- 2 servings of rice, boiled
- 2 containers of baby spinach

Step By Step Instructions for Recipe:
1. Prepare a griddle for medium cooking.
2. Peppers and zucchini should be cut thinly and then mixed with olive oil, garlic powder, salt, and pepper.
3. Cook the chicken breasts on the grill for about 6 minutes total, 5 on each side.
4. Cook the veggies for 2–3 minutes per side on a hot grill until caramelized and tender.
5. Split the rice and baby greens between two serving dishes. Cut up some chicken breasts and throw them in there.
6. Before serving, sprinkle on the cooked veggies.

Nutritional Analysis: Quantity of Energy in Calories: 515, Quantity of Protein: 47g, Quantity of Carbs: 42g, Quantity of Fat: 18g, Quantity of Fiber: 7g

45. Salmon Salad

Making and Duration Time: 13 minutes
Cooking Duration: 12-16 minutes **Number of Portions:** 2

Required Material for this Recipe:
- Two pieces of fish (salmon)
- Approximately one tablespoon of olive oil
- Four servings of mixed salad vegetables
- One-third of a cup of sliced cherry tomatoes
- Red onion, diced, 1/4 cup
- 1/4 cup of cucumber slices
- Fresh cilantro, minced (about 2 teaspoons)
- Lemon juice, about 2 teaspoons
- 2 tablespoons of honey, 2 tablespoons of Dijon mustard
- One-fourth cup of olive oil
- Pepper and salt

Step By Step Instructions for Recipe:
1. Turn the oven on to 400 degrees.
2. The salmon pieces need to be salted and peppered.

3. In an oven-safe skillet, heat up 1 spoonful of olive oil over medium heat.
4. The salmon pieces should be added and cooked for about 3 minutes on each side.
5. The fish should be done after 8-10 minutes in the oven.
6. Mixed salad, cherry tomatoes, red onion, cucumber, and cilantro should be tossed.
7. Mix together the honey, Dijon mustard, lemon juice, and olive oil for the sauce.
8. Split the salad between two dishes, then place a salmon piece on top of each. Serve.

Nutritional Analysis: Quantity of Energy in Calories: 506, Quantity of Protein: 33g, Quantity of Carbs: 16g, Quantity of Fat: 37g, Quantity of Fiber: 4g

45. Chickpea and Avocado Salad

Making and Duration Time: 11 minutes
Number of Portions: 2

Required Material for this Recipe:
- One can of legumes (chickpeas) drained and washed.
- Diced, mature avocado; one
- Half a cucumber and half a red onion, sliced
- Pepper, hot, 1/2 cup chopped
- Fresh cilantro, minced; 1 fistful
- Olive oil, enough for two teaspoons
- The juice of two lemons, measured in tablespoons
- Pepper and salt

Step By Step Instructions for Recipe:
1. Put the chickpeas, avocado, onion, cucumber, bell pepper, and cilantro in a dish and mix well.
2. Olive oil, lemon juice, salt, and pepper are the vinaigrette ingredients.
3. Toss the lettuce with the vinaigrette after it has been drizzled over it.
4. To serve, divide the salad among dishes.

Nutritional Analysis: Quantity of Energy in Calories: 402, Quantity of Protein: 12g, Quantity of Fat: 26g, Quantity of Carbs: 36g, Quantity of Fiber: 16g

46. Turmeric and Ginger Chicken Stir-Fry

Making and Duration Time: 13 minutes **Cooking Duration:** 15 minutes **Number of Portions:** 4

Required Material for this Recipe:
- Approximately two tablespoons of coconut oil
- Chicken breasts, skinless and boneless, weighing one pound
- An onion, cut in half
- Tender bell peppers, cut
- One cup of broccoli buds
- Mushrooms, cut, one cup
- Minced ginger, 1 tablespoon
- Garlic, chopped, 1 tablespoon
- One teaspoon of ground turmeric
- A pinch of black pepper and salt
- One-fourth cup of minced fresh coriander

Step By Step Instructions for Recipe:
1. Coconut oil should be warmed over medium heat in a skillet or griddle.
2. Place the poultry inside and roast for 5 to 7 minutes, or until it is golden.
3. Throw in some chopped onion, pepper, broccoli, and mushrooms and pop the skillet in the oven for 5–7 minutes.
4. Combine the salt, black pepper, turmeric, ginger, and garlic in a skillet and stir.
5. Keep everything in the pan for another minute or two until the chicken is done and the veggies have absorbed the seasonings.
6. Serve heated, garnished with fresh cilantro.

Nutritional Analysis: Quantity of Energy in Calories: 241, Quantity of Protein: 25g, Quantity of Fat: 11g, Quantity of Carbs: 11g, Quantity of Fiber: 3g

47. Quinoa and Black Bean Bowl

Making and Duration Time: 10 minutes **Cooking Duration:** 20 minutes **Number of Portions:** 4

Required Material for this Recipe:
- Uncooked quinoa equals one cup.
- Black beans from a can, strained and washed

- One scarlet bell pepper, sliced
- One avocado, sliced
- Juice of one citrus
- 2 teaspoons olive oil
- Just 1 tsp cumin
- Pepper and salt

Step By Step Instructions for Recipe:
1. Follow the package instructions for cooking quinoa.
2. The quinoa, black beans, red bell pepper, and avocado should all be mixed together in a dish after cooking.
3. Lime juice, olive oil, powdered cumin, salt, and pepper should all be mixed together in a dish.
4. Toss the quinoa and legume combination after adding the sauce to ensure everything is evenly distributed.
5. Prepare and serve right away, or cool and save for later.

Nutritional Analysis: Quantity of Energy in Calories: 329, Quantity of Fat: 13g, Carbohydrate: 44g, Quantity of Fiber: 12g, Quantity of Protein: 12

48. Mediterranean Salad with Roasted Chicken

Making and Duration Time: 12 minutes **Cooking Duration:** 15 minutes **Number of Portions:** 4

Required Material for this Recipe:
- 2 poultry breasts, deboned and skinless
- One-fourth cup of olive oil
- 1/4 cup of fresh lemon juice
- Dried oregano, one teaspoon
- Pepper and salt
- Four servings of vegetable salad
- Half a pound of immature tomatoes, sliced
- Kalamata olives, 1/2 cup
- feta cheese, shredded (about 1/2 cup)

Step By Step Instructions for Recipe:
1. Preheat a barbecue skillet on the stovetop.
2. Olive oil, lemon juice, dried oregano, salt, and pepper should all be mixed together in a dish.
3. Put the chicken breasts in a small bowl and pour the marinade over them. Ten minutes

of marinating time is recommended for the poultry.

4. Chicken should be grilled for 6–8 minutes per side, or until an internal temperature of 165 degrees is reached.

5. Put the feta cheese, cherry tomatoes, Kalamata olives, and mixed leaves in a dish and toss them together. Grilled poultry can be easily sliced and added to a salad.

6. Combine all ingredients by tossing them together, then serve.

Nutritional Analysis: Quantity of Energy in Calories: 373, Quantity of Fat: 27g, Carbohydrate: 10g, Quantity of Fiber: 2g, Quantity of Protein: 23g

49. Small Sweet Potato and Black Bean Tacos

Making and Duration Time: 15 minutes **Cooking Duration:** 30 minutes **Number of Portions:** 4

Required Material for this Recipe:
- Cut up 4 tiny, sweet potatoes and skin them.
- A tablespoon of olive oil
- Ground cumin, 1 teaspoon
- Smoked paprika, 12 teaspoons
- a pinch of red pepper flakes
- 1/4 teaspoon of salt

- Black beans, strained and washed from one 15-ounce can
- One-fourth cup of freshly cut parsley
- 2 Tablespoons of Pure Lime Juice
- Eight maize tacos.
- One sliced avocado

Step By Step Instructions for Recipe:
1. Preheat oven to 400 degrees Fahrenheit, baking sheet covered in parchment paper.
2. Olive oil, cumin, paprika, chili pepper, and salt should be mixed together and then tossed with the sweet potatoes.
3. Spread the sweet potatoes in a single line on the oven sheet. Tender and faintly caramelized after 20 to 25 minutes of cooking.
4. In another dish, mix together the black beans, parsley, and lime juice.
5. The tortillas can be heated on the griddle or in the oven.
6. Put some of the black bean combinations in the bottom of each tortilla, then add some baked sweet potato and sliced avocado. Serve.

Nutritional Analysis: Quantity of Energy in Calories: 362, Quantity of Protein: 9g, Quantity of Fat: 12g, Quantity of Carbs: 58g, Quantity of Fiber: 15g.

CHAPTER 5: DINNER RECIPES

50. Baked Salmon with Vegetables

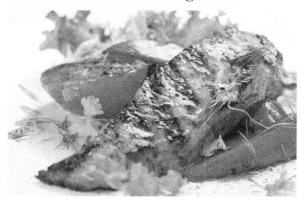

Making and Duration Time: 13 minutes
Cooking Duration: 20-25 minutes **Number of Portions:** 2

Required Material for this Recipe:
- Two pieces of fish, Salmon
- Vegetables, about two tablespoons (e.g., zucchini, bell peppers, cherry tomatoes)
- Two garlic bulbs, chopped
- 1/4 teaspoon of salt
- 1/4 teaspoon of pepper
- Olive oil, 2 tablespoons
- Parsley minced; 1 tablespoon

Step By Step Instructions for Recipe:
1. Turn the oven on to 400 degrees.
2. Prepare a roasting dish for the fish pieces and vegetables.
3. Olive oil, salt, pepper, and chopped garlic should be mixed. Spread the oil concoction over the fish and vegetables.
4. Put everything in the oven and simmer for 20–25 minutes, or until the fish is done and the veggies are tender.
5. Sprinkle some newly chopped parsley on top before serving.

Nutritional Analysis: Quantity of Energy in Calories: 435, Total Quantity of Fat: 28g, Quantity of Carbs: 11g, Quantity of Fiber: 3g, Quantity of Protein: 36g

51. Chickpea Stew with Spinach

Making and Duration Time: 15 minutes
Cooking Duration: 30 minutes **Number of Portions:** 4

Required Material for this Recipe:
- One 15-ounce can of chickpeas, drained and washed
- An Onion, Diced
- Two garlic bulbs, chopped
- Vegetable stock, two cups
- Spinach, minced, two tablespoons
- Tomatoes, diced (1 cup)
- 1/2 tsp coriander
- Paprika, one spoonful
- Turmeric, half a teaspoon
- Approximately 1/2 tsp. of salt and 1/4 tsp. of pepper
- Olive oil, enough for 2 teaspoons

Step By Step Instructions for Recipe:
1. Olive oil should be warmed over medium heat in a big saucepan.
2. Throw in some garlic and onions and cook them until they're aromatic and tender.
3. Stir in the coriander, paprika, turmeric, salt, and pepper along with the chickpeas, vegetable stock, shredded spinach, and tomatoes.
4. For tender veggies, bring the broth to a boil, then reduce heat and cook for 25-30 minutes.
5. Keep warm.

Nutritional Analysis: Quantity of Energy in Calories: 220kcal, Quantity of Fat: 9g, Quantity of Carbs: 28g, Quantity of Protein: 9g, Quantity of Fiber: 7g

52. Grilled Salmon with Avocado Salsa and Lime

Making and Duration Time: 11 minutes
Cooking Duration: 10 minutes **Number of Portions:** 4

Required Material for this Recipe:
- Four salmon pieces
- Pepper and salt
- Olive oil, enough for 2 teaspoons
- Two sliced mature avocados
- A bit of red scallion, chopped
- Pepper, hot, sliced
- To 1 lime juice.
- One-fourth cup of freshly cut parsley

Step By Step Instructions for Recipe:
1. Prepare a medium fire in the griddle.
2. Season the salmon pieces with salt and pepper and rub with olive oil.
3. Salmon takes about 5 minutes per side on the grill.
4. Mix the chopped avocado, onion, and bell pepper together. Combine lime juice and parsley and stir to combine.
5. Serve the seared salmon with a dollop of avocado sauce.

Nutritional Analysis: Quantity of Energy in Calories: 420kcal, Quantity of Fat: 28g, Quantity of Protein: 34g, Quantity of Carbs: 11g, Quantity of Fiber: 7g

53. Grilled Salmon with Cauliflower and Broccoli Rice

Making and Duration Time: 11 minutes
Cooking Duration: 15 minutes **Number of Portions:** 4

Required Material for this Recipe:
- Four salmon fillets
- Two Tablespoons of Olive Oil
- Chopped garlic, 2
- Spice and seasoning
- One broccoli bundle
- Cauliflower, enough for one cup
- Two teaspoons of finely chopped fresh parsley
- Putting out lemon wedges

Step By Step Instructions for Recipe:
1. Preheat the griddle to medium.
2. Put the olive oil, garlic, salt, and pepper in a bowl and mix.
3. Apply the olive oil combination by drizzling it over the salmon pieces.
4. Cook the fish on a hot grill for about 5–7 minutes per side.
5. The broccoli and cauliflower should be processed in a food processor until a rice-like consistency is reached.
6. Put some olive oil in a big pan and cook it over medium heat.
7. Cook the cauliflower, broccoli, and rice for about 5 minutes, or until the vegetables are soft.
8. The cauliflower-broccoli rice would benefit from a sprinkle of fresh minced cilantro.
9. Place lemon slices on the side and serve with seared fish, cauliflower rice, and asparagus.

Nutritional Analysis: Quantity of Energy in Calories: 305, Quantity of Protein: 29g, Quantity of Carbs: 9g, Quantity of Fat: 18g, Quantity of Fiber: 4g

54. Grilled Salmon & Mango Salsa

Making and Duration Time: 15 minutes
Cooking Duration: 11 minutes **Number of Portions:** 4

Required Material for this Recipe:
- Mango, one, skinned and sliced
- Four salmon pieces (6 ounces each)
- 1/4 teaspoon of salt
- A Pinch of Pepper
- A quarter cup of chopped red scallion
- One-fourth cup of minced fresh coriander
- Lime juice, one teaspoonful
- Two teaspoons of butter

Step By Step Instructions for Recipe:
1. Start up the griddle at medium heat.
2. The salmon pieces need to be salted and peppered.
3. Salmon pieces need about 4–5 minutes on the grill per side to roast through.
4. While the salmon is in the oven, whip up a batch of mango sauce. Dice the mango and

add it to the dish with the red onion, parsley, lime juice, and olive oil.

5. Mango sauce should be served alongside broiled fish.

Nutritional Analysis: Quantity of Energy in Calories: 280, Quantity of Fat: 13g, Quantity of Carbs: 8g, Quantity of Fiber: 1g, Quantity of Protein: 31g

55. Grilled Salmon with Garlic and Fresh Herbs

Making and Duration Time: 11 minutes **Cooking Duration:** 15 minutes **Number of Portions:** 4

Required Material for this Recipe:
- Four 6-ounce chunks of salmon
- Four garlic bulbs, chopped
- One-fourth cup of fresh herbs, minced (such as parsley, thyme, and dill)
- Two teaspoons of butter
- Pepper and salt
- Sliced lemons

Step By Step Instructions for Recipe:
1. Get the griddle hot, but not too hot.
2. Toss olive oil, spices, and garlic together.
3. Rub the herb combination onto the salmon pieces after seasoning them with salt and pepper.
4. Cook salmon pieces for about 5–7 minutes per side, starting with the skin side down.
5. Accompany with lemon slices when serving.

Nutritional Analysis: Quantity of Energy in Calories: 285, Quantity of Protein: 36g, Quantity of Fat: 13g, Quantity of Carbs: 1g, Quantity of Fiber: 0g

56. Grilled Salmon with Ginger-Turmeric Gravy

Making and Duration Time: 13 minutes **Cooking Duration:** 17 minutes **Number of Portions:** 4

Required Material for this Recipe:
- Salmon pieces. (6 ounces each)
- Approximately one tablespoon of olive oil

- Pepper and salt
- Two teaspoons of ground cinnamon
- Turmeric, 1 tbsp
- two tablespoons of honey
- Add 2 tablespoons of low-sodium soy sauce
- Rice vinegar, 2 tbsp
- Water, 2 tablespoons worth

Step By Step Instructions for Recipe:
1. Prepare a medium fire in the griddle.
2. Season the salmon pieces with salt and pepper and rub them with olive oil.
3. Salmon should be prepared for 5–6 minutes per side.
4. Soy sauce, rice vinegar, water, ginger, turmeric, honey should all be whisked together.
5. Drizzle the ginger-turmeric marinade over the top of the cooked fish and serve.

Nutritional Analysis: Quantity of Energy in Calories: 300, Quantity of Fat: 17g, Quantity of Carbs: 9g, Quantity of Fiber: 1g, Quantity of Protein: 28g

57. Grilled Salmon with Quinoa and Grilled Veggies

Making and Duration Time: 15 minutes **Cooking Duration:** 27 minutes **Number of Portions:** 4

Required Material for this Recipe:
- Four salmon pieces (About 6 ounces each)
- One cup of quinoa
- Vegetable stock, two pints
- One courgette, cut.
- One scarlet bell pepper, cut
- One golden onion, cut
- Olive oil, 2 tablespoons
- A single teaspoon of dried garlic
- Basil, desiccated, 1 teaspoon
- Pepper and salt

Step By Step Instructions for Recipe:
1. Preheat the oven to 425 degrees.
2. After a quick rinse, put the quinoa in a saucepan with the vegetable stock.
3. Get it boiling, then turn it down and let it stew for about 15 minutes.

4. Mix the cut vegetables with olive oil, and seasonings (salt, pepper, garlic powder, and chopped basil).
5. Roast in the oven at 400 degrees for 20–25 minutes, or until fork-tender.
6. Grill the salmon pieces for about 4 to 6 minutes per side, or until done, while you prepare the veggies.
7. Prepare quinoa and grilled veggies to accompany the fish.

Nutritional Analysis: Quantity of Energy in Calories: 473, Quantity of Protein: 39g, Quantity of Fat: 23g, Quantity of Carbs: 31g, Quantity of Fiber: 5g

58. Grilled Salmon and Veggies

Making and Duration Time: 13 minutes **Cooking Duration:** 17 minutes **Number of Portions:** 4

Required Material for this Recipe:
- Here are your four salmon pieces (6 ounces each)
- One courgetti cut
- 1 chopped golden squash
- Sliced red bell pepper (1 pepper)
- Two teaspoons of butter
- Pepper and salt
- 1 cut citrus
- Garnish with chopped fresh cilantro

Step By Step Instructions for Recipe:

1. Heat the griddle to a comfortable level.
2. Mix together olive oil, bell pepper, and squash, then season with salt and pepper.
3. Salmon pieces need about 5–6 minutes of cooking time per side.
4. Grill the lemon slices for the final two minutes.
5. barbecue the veggies for 5–7 minutes, depending on their size, in a barbecue pan or aluminum foil dish.
6. Place cooked veggies and lemon wedges atop the fish before serving.
7. Fresh cilantro for garnish

Nutritional Analysis: Quantity of Energy in Calories: 345, Quantity of Fat: 22g, Quantity of Protein: 31g, Quantity of Carbs: 7g, Quantity of Fiber: 2g

59. Lemon Salmon with Asparagus

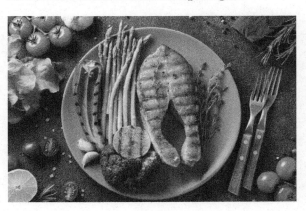

Making and Duration Time: 11 minutes **Cooking Duration:** 20 minutes **Number of Portions:** 4

Required Material for this Recipe:
- Here are your four salmon pieces.
- Asparagus with the tips snapped off
- Three cloves of chopped garlic
- Lemon, cut, 1
- Olive oil, enough for two teaspoons
- Pepper and salt

Step By Step Instructions for Recipe:

1. Preheat the oven to 375 degrees.
2. Place the salmon pieces and asparagus in a roasting tray.
3. Salt and pepper the fish and asparagus before pouring the olive oil over the top.
4. Sprinkle the minced garlic on top of the fish.
5. Accompany the fish with a stack of lemon segments.
6. Cook for 20 minutes, flipping once, until the salmon is done and the asparagus is tender.
7. Serve.

Nutritional Analysis: Quantity of Energy in Calories: 329, Quantity of Fat: 19g, Quantity of Protein: 35g, Quantity of Carbs: 5g, Quantity of Fiber: 2g

60. Lemon Garlic Shrimp and Broccoli Sautéed

Making and Duration Time: 13 minutes **Cooking Duration:** 11 minutes **Number of Portions:** 2

Required Material for this Recipe:
- Raw shrimp, one pound, skinned and deveined
- Broccoli flower buds, 2 cups
- Two hands full of chopped garlic
- Olive oil, enough for two teaspoons
- 1/4 glass of lemon juice
- Pepper and salt

Step By Step Instructions for Recipe:
1. Olive oil should be warmed over medium heat in a skillet.
2. In a skillet, combine the shrimp, garlic, and olive oil. Bake for 2–3 minutes, or until the prawns turn rosy.
3. Add the broccoli and boil for 2–3 minutes, occasionally stirring, until it is soft.
4. Season the prawns and asparagus with salt and pepper, and then add the juice of half a lemon. Keep warm.

Nutritional Analysis: Quantity of Energy in Calories: 347, Quantity of Fat: 18g, Quantity of Carbs: 14g, Quantity of Fiber: 4g, Quantity of Protein: 35g

61. Mediterranean Chicken Skewers

Making and Duration Time: 15 minutes **Cooking Duration:** 17 minutes **Number of Portions:** 4

Required Material for this Recipe:
- Cut up four boneless, skinless chicken breasts.
- Pepper, red, minced: one, diced
- One sliced golden bell pepper
- One sliced scarlet onion
- Exactly one courgette, diced
- One-fourth cup of olive oil
- Lemon juice, 2 tablespoons
- Oregano, powdered, one teaspoon
- Thyme, powdered, one sprinkle

- Smoked paprika, 1/2 tsp
- Pepper and salt

Step By Step Instructions for Recipe:
1. Prepare a medium fire in the griddle.
2. Olive oil, lemon juice, oregano, dried thyme, smoky paprika, salt, and pepper should be mixed together.
3. In a dish, combine the poultry, marinate, red onion, red bell pepper, yellow bell pepper, and zucchini.
4. Prepare spears with poultry and veggies.
5. Cook the chicken kebabs on a griddle for 10–12 minutes, flipping them once or twice.

Nutritional Analysis: Quantity of Energy in Calories: 326, Quantity of Fat: 19g, Quantity of Protein: 30g, Quantity of Carbs: 10g, Quantity of Fiber: 3g

62. One Pan Baked Salmon and Zucchini

Making and Duration Time: 7 minutes **Cooking Duration:** 17 minutes **Number of Portions:** 2

Required Material for this Recipe:
- Two pieces of fish, Salmon
- Two teaspoons of olive oil
- 2 small zucchinis
- Pepper and salt
- One cut lemon, One teaspoon of powdered dill

Step By Step Instructions for Recipe:
1. Turn the oven on to 400 degrees.
2. Prepare a roasting sheet by arranging the salmon pieces and zucchini on it.
3. Season the fish and asparagus with salt, pepper, and chopped dill, then drizzle with olive oil and serve.
4. Salmon pieces should have lemon segments atop them.
5. If you want your fish done through and your zucchini soft and delicate, a 12- to 15-minute bake time is perfect.
6. Keep warm

Nutritional Analysis: Quantity of Energy in Calories: 362, Quantity of Fat: 22g, Quantity of Carbs: 8g, Quantity of Fiber: 4g, Quantity of Protein: 34g

63. Quinoa and Black Bean Stuffed Bell Peppers

Making and Duration Time: 18 minutes
Cooking Duration: 45 minutes **Number of Portions:** 4

Required Material for this Recipe:
- 4 scarlet bell peppers, halved and seeded
- Olive oil, 1 tablespoon
- One small shallot, minced
- Two chopped garlic
- Rinsed rice equals one cup.
- Low-sodium vegetable broth, two pints
- A pinch of coriander
- Pepper and salt
- Smoked paprika, one teaspoon
- Chili powder, half a teaspoon
- Beans, black, from a can; strain and blanch
- Cherry tomatoes, half a cup
- One-fourth cup of minced fresh coriander

Step By Step Instructions for Recipe:

1. Preheat the oven to 375 degrees.
2. Bell peppers should be cut in half and placed in a roasting dish.
3. To soften the onion and garlic, warm the olive oil in a skillet over medium heat and add the two ingredients.
4. Mix in some chile pepper, coriander, smoky paprika, rice, and veggie stock.
5. Bring to a boil, then reduce heat to low and stew for 15–20 minutes, or until the liquid is consumed and the quinoa is tender.
6. Sprinkle some salt and pepper on top, then add the result beans, cherry tomatoes, and parsley.
7. Cover the pepper halves with the rice concoction.
8. Cook the dish, covered with foil, for 25-30 minutes, or until the peppers are tender, whichever comes first.

Nutritional Analysis: Quantity of Energy in Calories: 321, Quantity of Fat: 8g, Quantity of Carbs: 52g, Quantity of Fiber: 14g, Quantity of Protein: 14g

64. Quinoa and Chickpea Stew with Paprika

Making and Duration Time: 13 minutes
Cooking Duration: 20 to 30 minutes **Number of Portions:** 4

Required Material for this Recipe:
- Two teaspoons of butter
- 1 medium onion, chopped 2 cloves of garlic, minced
- 1 teaspoon of cumin seed
- 1 teaspoon of cilantro powder
- a pinch of smoky paprika
- a pinch of red pepper flakes
- One 14-ounce can have chopped tomatoes
- 1 (15 oz.) can of legumes, drained and washed
- Vegetable broth, 2 pints
- Rinsed rice equals one cup.
- Pepper and salt
- Decorative fresh parsley, 2 tablespoons

Step By Step Instructions for Recipe:

1. Olive oil should be heated in a pan over medium heat.
2. Cook the onion and garlic until the onion is tender, stirring occasionally.
3. Toss in the chili, smoky paprika, cumin powder, and cilantro.
4. Stir in the chopped tomatoes, vegetable broth, rice, and beans.
5. Bring everything to a boil, then reduce heat to low and let stew cook for 25–30 minutes, or until quinoa is tender and the stew has thickened.
6. Season with salt and pepper and garnish with minced fresh parsley before serving.

Nutritional Analysis: Quantity of Energy in Calories: 345, Quantity of Fat: 7g, Quantity of Carbs: 58g, Quantity of Fiber: 12g, Quantity of Protein: 13g

65. Quinoa Stuffed Bell Peppers

Making and Duration Time: 20 minutes
Cooking Duration: 40 minutes **Number of Portions:** 4

Required Material for this Recipe:
- Four bell peppers, cut in half and seasoned
- One cup of ready-to-eat rice
- Black beans from a can, strained and washed
- One tiny, finely minced scallion
- Two garlic bulbs, chopped
- Cumin, one teaspoon
- A pinch of paprika
- A pinch of cayenne pepper flakes
- 1/4 teaspoon of salt
- black pepper, 1/4 teaspoons
- One-fourth cup of freshly cut parsley
- Shredded cheddar cheese equaling 1/4 cup

Step By Step Instructions for Recipe:
1. Preheat the oven to 375 degrees.
2. Onion and garlic should be cooked until soft over medium heat.
3. Cooked quinoa, black beans, cumin, paprika, cayenne pepper, salt, black pepper, and cilantro should be added to the pan and tossed together until everything is evenly distributed.
4. Place the cut bell peppers in a roasting dish.
5. Stuff the rice and black bean combination into the bell pepper halves.
6. Cover the dish with foil and bake for 25-30 minutes.
7. Remove the paper and sprinkle the grated cheddar over the bell peppers.
8. Continue cooking for another 10 minutes, or until the cheese is melted and frothing.
9. Serve.

Nutritional Analysis: Quantity of Energy in Calories: 272, Quantity of Fat: 7g, Quantity of Protein: 14g, Quantity of Carbs: 43g, Quantity of Fiber: 13g

66. Quinoa and Veggie Sauté

Making and Duration Time: 15 minutes
Cooking Duration: 21 minutes **Number of Portions:** 4

Required Material for this Recipe:
- A cup of quinoa, after being washed and drained
- The equivalent of two glasses of water
- Two teaspoons of butter
- Two bulbs of chopped garlic
- One scarlet bell pepper, cut
- One golden bell pepper, cut
- One courgette, cut.
- Squash, golden, one, cut
- Mushrooms, cut, one cup
- one-fourth cup of minced basil
- Pepper and salt

Step By Step Instructions for Recipe:
1. Put the quinoa and water in a pot and bring to a simmer. After the water has been drained and the quinoa is soft, it is time to turn down the heat, cover it, and let it boil for 15 to 20 minutes.
2. Cook the garlic in the olive oil for 30 seconds over medium heat until it browns.
3. Throw in some mushrooms, peppers, zucchini, and squash, and roast at 400 for 10 minutes.
4. Dress with salt and pepper, stir in some minced basil, and serve well heat.

Nutritional Analysis: Quantity of Energy in Calories: 223, Quantity of Protein: 8g, Quantity of Fat: 7g, Quantity of Carbs: 36g, Quantity of Fiber: 6g

67. Spicy Turkey and Soft Potato

Making and Duration Time: 13 minutes
Cooking Duration: 23 minutes **Number of Portions:** 4

Required Material for this Recipe:
- One pound of poultry meat, Turkey
- Two potatoes, average in size, skinned and diced
- Sweet pepper, rot
- The golden onion is chopped.
- Two bulbs of chopped garlic

- Olive oil, 1 tablespoon
- Paprika, 1 teaspoon
- Cumin, half a teaspoon
- 1/4 teaspoon pepper, the same quantity of cayenne pepper

Step By Step Instructions for Recipe:

1. Olive oil should be warmed over medium heat in a skillet. Ground turkey should be added and simmered for about 5–7 minutes.
2. Mix in the sweet potatoes, peppers, onions, garlic, paprika, salt, black pepper, cumin, and cayenne.
3. Cover the skillet and reduce the heat to medium. Tender potatoes can be achieved after 10 to 15 minutes in the oven.
4. Bring the heated pan of poultry and potatoes to the table.

Nutritional Analysis: Quantity of Energy in Calories: 290, Quantity of Fat: 12g, Quantity of Carbs: 20g, Quantity of Fiber: 4g, Quantity of Protein: 26g

68. Turmeric Chicken Sauté with Dark Rice

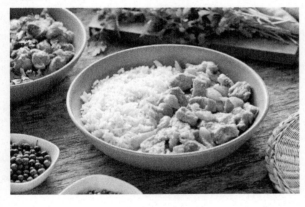

Making and Duration Time: 17 minutes **Cooking Duration:** 25 minutes **Number of Portions:** 4

Required Material for this Recipe:

- Chicken breasts without the bone and flesh, weighed at 1 pound
- Brown rice, two servings
- Water, 4 mugs
- Pepper, rot, cut, one
- 1 golden bell pepper, cut
- Onion, chopped, one

- Coconut oil, two teaspoons
- Ginger, minced, 1 teaspoonful
- Two garlic bulbs, chopped
- Turmeric powder, one teaspoonful
- Pepper and salt

Step By Step Instructions for Recipe:

1. Brown rice, after being washed, is added to water in a pot.
2. To cook, bring to a boil, then reduce heat and stew for 20–25 minutes.
3. Coconut oil should be warmed in a skillet over medium heat. Chicken pieces should be stir-fried for about 5–6 minutes.
4. Stir-fry the onion and bell pepper segments for three to four minutes.
5. In a mixing bowl, combine the shredded ginger, chopped garlic, powdered turmeric, salt, and pepper.
6. Brown rice should be served under stir-fry.

Nutritional Analysis: Quantity of Energy in Calories: 426, Quantity of Protein: 32g, Quantity of Fat: 9g, Quantity of Carbs: 56g, Quantity of Fiber: 6g

69. Turmeric Chicken & Roasted Veggies

Making and Duration Time: 11 minutes **Cooking Duration:** 30 minutes **Number of Portions:** 4

Required Material for this Recipe:

- Four poultry breasts without the bones and flesh
- Approximately one tablespoon of olive oil
- Turmeric, 1 teaspoon
- Paprika, 1/2 tsp
- a pinch of dried garlic
- Pepper and salt
- One large, sweet potato, skinned and diced.
- One scarlet bell pepper, sliced
- One golden bell pepper, sliced
- One small red scallion, sliced
- Parsley, minced, two teaspoons

Step By Step Instructions for Recipe:

1. Turn the oven on to 400 degrees.
2. Combine the olive oil, spices, salt, pepper, and garlic powder.
3. The seasoning combination should be sprinkled over the poultry breasts.

4. The chicken breasts should be baked in a roasting tray.
5. Chop up some potatoes, peppers, and onions, and throw them all together in a dish with some olive oil, salt, and pepper.
6. Put the poultry in a roasting tray and surround it with the veggies.
7. Chicken should be done in 25-30 minutes, and veggies should be tender.
8. Garnish the poultry and veggies with minced fresh parsley before serving.

Nutritional Analysis: Quantity of Energy in Calories: 277, Quantity of Protein: 30g, Quantity of Carbs: 20g, Quantity of Fat: 8g, Quantity of Fiber: 4g

70. Turmeric Chicken Breasts & Quinoa

Making and Duration Time: 13 minutes **Cooking Duration:** 30 minutes **Number of Portions:** 4

Required Material for this Recipe:
- Four poultry breasts without the bones and flesh
- Olive oil, enough for two teaspoons
- Two teaspoons of turmeric
- A dash of paprika
- Powdered garlic, one teaspoon
- Just a pinch of salt
- a pinch of spice
- Rinsed quinoa equals one cup
- Approximately one-fourth cup of minced cilantro
- a single lemon, segmented
- Chicken broth, 2 mugs

Step By Step Instructions for Recipe:
1. Preheat the oven to 375 degrees.
2. Combine olive oil with the spice's turmeric, paprika, smoked paprika, garlic powder, salt, and pepper.
3. Before putting them on a roasting pan, rub the poultry breasts with the seasoning combination.
4. To prepare the poultry, put it in the microwave for 25 to 30 minutes.
5. Cook the rice in a pot with the chicken broth while the poultry is in the oven. Cook for 15–20 minutes at a low simmer

after bringing to a boil for the liquid to be consumed and the quinoa to be prepared.
6. Sprinkle the rice with minced cilantro and top with the chicken; serve with lemon wedges.

Nutritional Analysis: Quantity of Energy in Calories: 375, Quantity of Fat: 10g, Quantity of Protein: 45g, Quantity of Carbs: 26g, Quantity of Fiber: 3g

71. Turmeric and Ginger Chicken with Soft Potatoes and Broccoli

Making and Duration Time: 15 minutes **Cooking Duration:** 45 minutes **Number of Portions:** 4

Required Material for this Recipe:
- Four poultry legs with bones
- One tablespoon of ground turmeric
- Ginger, minced, 1 tablespoon
- Olive oil, 1 tablespoon
- Just a pinch of salt
- Two sweet potatoes, about average in size, skinned and sliced
- Broccoli flower buds, 2 cups
- Two garlic bulbs, chopped
- Two teaspoons of honey

Step By Step Instructions for Recipe:
1. Preheat the oven to 375 degrees.
2. Combine the ginger, turmeric, olive oil, and salt in a bowl.
3. Apply the turmeric paste to the poultry legs.
4. Throw the legs of poultry into a roasting tray.
5. Throw in some sweet potatoes, some broccoli, and some chopped garlic.
6. Honey should be drizzled on top.
7. Allow 45 minutes of cooking time to ensure the poultry is fully prepared and the vegetables are succulent. Serve

Nutritional Analysis: Quantity of Energy in Calories: 404, Quantity of Fat: 16g, Quantity of Protein: 29g, Quantity of Carbs: 36g, Quantity of Fiber: 6g

72. Baked Salmon with Grilled Veggies

Making and Duration Time: 13 minutes **Cooking Duration:** 20-25 minutes **Number of Portions:** 2

Required Material for this Recipe:
- Two pieces of fish, Salmon
- One tiny, sweet potato, scraped and diced
- One red bell pepper seeded and cut.
- A single tiny golden squash, cut
- One tiny zucchini, cut.
- Two teaspoons of butter
- An Equivalent of One-Half of a Teaspoon of Garlic
- Pepper and salt

Step By Step Instructions for Recipe:
1. Turn the oven on to 400 degrees.
2. Mix the squashes, peppers, and zucchini with olive oil, garlic powder, salt, and pepper.
3. Prepare a roasting tray by spreading the veggies out in a uniform line.
4. Put it in the oven and turn it on to bake for 10 minutes.
5. Take the baking tray out of the oven and put the pieces of salmon on it.
6. Cook the fish with salt and pepper.
7. Put the fish in the oven and bake for 10–15 minutes. Serve.

Nutritional Analysis: Quantity of Energy in Calories: 360, Quantity of Fat: 17g, Quantity of Carbs: 17g, Quantity of Fiber: 4g, Quantity of Protein: 35g

73. Turkey and Vegetable Sauté

Making and Duration Time: 13 minutes **Cooking Duration:** 10 minutes **Number of Portions:** 2

Required Material for this Recipe:
- 1/2 pound of ground turkey
- Two teaspoons of butter
- One tiny onion, diced.
- One red bell pepper seeded and cut.
- One tiny zucchini, cut.
- One tiny golden squash, cut

- Powdered garlic, half a teaspoon
- Ground ginger, 1/2 teaspoon
- Pepper and salt

Step By Step Instructions for Recipe:
1. Olive oil should be heated in a skillet over medium heat.
2. Put the ground turkey in the oven and roast it until it's golden.
3. Combine the onions, peppers, zucchini, and squash and pour them into the pot.
4. Put in some salt, pepper, powdered ginger, and garlic powder.
5. The veggies will be ready after 5 minutes of sautéing. Serve.

Nutritional Analysis: Quantity of Energy in Calories: 281, Quantity of Fat: 15g, Quantity of Carbs: 12g, Quantity of Fiber: 3g, Quantity of Protein: 26g

74. Grilled Chicken with Lemon Garlic Marinade

Making and Duration Time: 11 minutes **Cooking Duration:** 12 to 15 minutes **Number of Portions:** 2

Required Material for this Recipe:
- Two chicken breasts without the skin and bones
- Olive oil, 2 tablespoons
- The extract from one citrus
- 1 minced garlic bulb
- Pepper and salt

Step By Step Instructions for Recipe:
1. In a dish, mix together the garlic, olive oil, lemon juice, salt, and pepper.
2. Place the poultry in a small baking dish and pour the marinate over top.
3. Refrigerate for at least 30 minutes and up to 4 hours while covered.
4. Prepare a medium fire in the griddle.
5. Cook the chicken breasts on a hot grill for about 7 minutes total (6 minutes per side). Serve.

Nutritional Analysis: Quantity of Energy in Calories: 260, Quantity of Fat: 14g, Quantity of Carbs: 2g, Quantity of Fiber: 0g, Quantity of Protein: 31g

CHAPTER 6: SIDE DISH RECIPES

75. Roasted Turmeric Cabbage

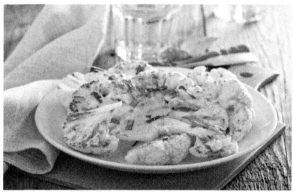

Making and Duration Time: 6 minutes **Cooking Duration:** 20 minutes **Number of Portions:** 4

Required Material for this Recipe:
- Several clusters of cauliflower from a whole head
- Two teaspoons of EVO oil
- Turmeric, crushed, a teaspoon
- Pepper and salt

Step By Step Instructions for Recipe:
1. Turn the oven on to 400 degrees.
2. Olive oil, powdered turmeric, salt, and pepper should be used to coat the cauliflower pieces.
3. Spread the broccoli out in a single layer on a baking tray.
4. To get them nice and soft and caramelized on the outside, roast them for 20 minutes. Keep warm

Nutritional Analysis: Quantity of Energy in Calories: 66, Quantity of Fat: 4g, Quantity of Carbs: 7g, Quantity of Fiber: 3g, Quantity of Protein: 3g

76. Lemon Roasted Brussels Sprouts with Garlic

Making and Duration Time: 10 minutes **Cooking Duration:** 25 minutes **Number of Portions:** 4

Required Material for this Recipe:
- Brussels sprouts, worth one pound, cleaned and cut in half
- Olive oil, 2 tablespoons
- Two minced garlic cloves
- One lemon's juice
- Pepper and salt

Step By Step Instructions for Recipe:
1. Turn the oven on to 400 degrees.
2. Olive oil, minced garlic, lemon juice, salt, and pepper should be combined with the Brussels sprouts.
3. Make sure there is only one stack of Brussels sprouts on the oven sheet.
4. For delicate, barely colored Brussels sprouts, roast them for 25 minutes.
5. Keep warm.

Nutritional Analysis: Quantity of Energy in Calories: 91, Quantity of Fat: 7g, Quantity of Carbs: 7g, Quantity of Fiber: 3g, Quantity of Protein: 3g

77. Balsamic Roasted Veggies

Making and Duration Time: 10 minutes **Cooking Duration:** 21 minutes **Number of Portions:** 4

Required Material for this Recipe:
- Two tablespoons of a variety of veggies, such as zucchini, onions, bell peppers, and mushrooms
- 2 tbsp of balsamic vinegar
- Olive oil, 1 tablespoon
- Dried oregano, 1 teaspoon
- Pepper and salt

Step By Step Instructions for Recipe:
1. Preheat the oven to 425 degrees.
2. After cleaning, cut the vegetables into small chunks for easier eating.
3. Whisk together the olive oil, balsamic vinegar, dried oregano, salt, and pepper.
4. Chop the veggies and spread them out on a baking sheet, then pour the vinegar concoction over them and stir to moisten them.
5. For 20 minutes, or until soft and beginning to color, place the veggies on a grill.

Nutritional Analysis: Quantity of Energy in Calories: 76, Quantity of Fat: 4g, Quantity of Carbs: 9g, Quantity of Fiber: 3g, Quantity of Protein: 2g

78. Lemon Quinoa with Garlic

Making and Duration Time: 7 minutes **Cooking Duration:** 17 minutes **Number of Portions:** 4

Required Material for this Recipe:
- Quinoa, one cup, drained.
- Two pints of stock made from vegetables
- Two teaspoons of butter
- Two bulbs of chopped garlic
- One lemon, squeezed and rind removed
- Pepper and salt
- sliced fresh cilantro

Step By Step Instructions for Recipe:
1. Olive oil should be warmed in a skillet over medium heat. Toss in the garlic, then roast for an additional minute or two until aromatic.
2. Stir the rice and veggie stock together in a skillet after it has been washed.
3. Achieve a simmer, then reduce the heat to medium and cover the pot.
4. Quinoa needs 15 minutes of cooking time to become soft and incorporate all of the cooking fluids.
5. Take it off the fire and season it with salt, pepper, lemon juice, and lemon zest. Add some minced fresh cilantro, and you're good to go.

Nutritional Analysis: Quantity of Energy in Calories: 160, Quantity of Fat: 4g, Quantity of Carbs: 26g, Quantity of Fiber: 3g, Quantity of Protein: 5g

79. Balsamic Grilled Brussels Sprouts

Making and Duration Time: 6 minutes **Cooking Duration:** 20-25 minutes **Number of Portions:** 4

Required Material for this Recipe:
- Belgian stems, one pound, halved
- Olive oil, enough for two teaspoons
- A splash of balsamic vinegar, or two teaspoons
- Powdered garlic, one teaspoon's worth
- Pepper and salt

Step By Step Instructions for Recipe:
1. Turn the oven on to 400 degrees.
2. Add balsamic vinegar, garlic powder, olive oil, salt, pepper, and Brussels sprouts, and mix well.
3. The Brussels sprouts should be spread out in a single line on a roasting tray.
4. Tender and caramelize for 20 to 25 minutes in the oven. Keep warm.

Nutritional Analysis: Quantity of Energy in Calories: 95, Quantity of Fat: 6.8g, Quantity of Carbs: 8.7g, Quantity of Fiber: 3.3g, Quantity of Protein: 2.9g

80. Lemon Asparagus & Garlic

Making and Duration Time: 7 minutes **Cooking Duration:** 10 minutes **Number of Portions:** 4

Required Material for this Recipe:
- Trim the ends off one pound of asparagus.
- Olive oil, enough for two teaspoons
- Two bulbs of chopped garlic
- Extract from one citrus, lemon
- Pepper and salt

Step By Step Instructions for Recipe:
1. Olive oil should be warmed over medium heat in a skillet.
2. Stirring continuously, put the chopped garlic in the oven, and roast for a minute.
3. Toss in the cleaned asparagus and roast for 5–7 minutes, tossing periodically, until the vegetable is soft and beginning to color.
4. Squeeze fresh lemon juice over the asparagus and season with salt and pepper right before serving.

Nutritional Analysis: Quantity of Energy in Calories: 70, Quantity of Fat: 5g, Quantity of Carbs: 5g, Quantity of Fiber: 2.5g, Quantity of Protein: 2.5g

81. Turmeric Grilled Carrots

Making and Duration Time: 4 minutes **Cooking Duration:** 25 minutes **Number of Portions:** 4

Required Material for this Recipe:
- Carrots, one pound, trimmed and sliced thinly.
- Olive oil, enough for two teaspoons
- A single spoonful of turmeric powder

- Pepper and salt

Step By Step Instructions for Recipe:
1. Turn the oven on to 400 degrees.
2. Olive oil, turmeric, salt, and pepper should all be combined with the carrots.
3. Carrots should be spread out in a single line on a roasting tray.
4. To achieve tenderness and browning in the oven, roast for 25 minutes. Keep warm.

Nutritional Analysis: Quantity of Energy in Calories: 85, Quantity of Fat: 5g, Quantity of Carbs: 10g, Quantity of Fiber: 3g, Quantity of Protein: 1g

82. Balsamic Roasted Carrots

Making and Duration Time: 7 minutes **Cooking Duration:** 25 minutes **Number of Portions:** 4

Required Material for this Recipe:
- Baby carrots and onions, one pound
- Olive oil, one tablespoon
- Balsamic vinegar, 1 teaspoonful
- Honey, one teaspoon
- Pepper and salt

Step By Step Instructions for Recipe:
1. Turn the oven on to 400 degrees.
2. Add honey, salt, pepper, balsamic vinegar, and olive oil to a bowl and mix well.
3. Toss in the tiny carrots and cover them thoroughly.
4. Spread the carrots out in a single line on a baking tray.
5. Put in the oven and roast for 20–25 minutes, or until soft. Quickly serve.

Nutritional Analysis: Quantity of Energy in Calories: 78, Quantity of Fat: 3.5g, Quantity of Carbs: 12g, Quantity of Fiber: 3g, Quantity of Protein: 1g

83. Broiled Asparagus with Parmesan Cheese and Lemon

Making and Duration Time: 6 minutes **Cooking Duration:** 10 minutes **Number of Portions:** 4

Required Material for this Recipe:
- One pound of asparagus, cut
- A tablespoon of olive oil.
- Juice from one lemon, 1 tbsp
- Parmesan cheese, shredded, 1/4 cup

- Pepper and salt

Step By Step Instructions for Recipe:
1. Get the griddle nice and toasty.
2. Put the asparagus in a dish and toss it with olive oil, lemon juice, salt, and pepper.
3. Prepare a baking tray with room for a single bed of asparagus.
4. Sprinkle some shredded Parmesan cheese over the asparagus.
5. To achieve a golden color and delicate texture, broil for 5–7 minutes. Quickly serve.

Nutritional Analysis: Quantity of Energy in Calories: 79, Quantity of Fat: 5g, Quantity of Carbs: 5g, Quantity of Fiber: 2g, Quantity of Protein: 6g

84. Cucumber Salad with Tomato

Making and Duration Time: 14 minutes **Number of Portions:** 4

Required Material for this Recipe:
- 2 cucumbers, trimmed and cut
- Tomatoes, 2 big, sliced
- Half of a chopped red scallion
- Chopped fresh parsley equaling 2 teaspoons
- Olive oil, enough for two teaspoons
- Red wine vinegar, one teaspoonful
- Pepper and salt

Step By Step Instructions for Recipe:
1. Combine the tomato and cucumber slices with the red onion and herbs.
2. In a small dish, whisk together the olive oil, red wine vinegar, salt, and pepper.
3. Toss the tomatoes and cucumbers in the dressing until everything is evenly distributed. Immediately serve.

Nutritional Analysis: Quantity of Energy in Calories: 93, Quantity of Fat: 7g, Quantity of Carbs: 7g, Quantity of Fiber: 2g, Quantity of Protein: 2g

85. Roasted Asparagus with Garlic

Making and Duration Time: 6 minutes **Cooking Duration:** 16 minutes **Number of Portions:** 4

Required Material for this Recipe:
- One pound of cut, fresh asparagus
- Two chopped garlic cloves

- There should be 1 tablespoon of olive oil
- Pepper and salt

Step By Step Instructions for Recipe:
1. Preheat the oven to 425 degrees.
2. Prepare a roasting tray for the asparagus.
3. Olive oil and chopped garlic should be drizzled and distributed on top.
4. Sprinkle some salt and pepper on it.
5. Put in the oven for 15 minutes at 400 degrees until soft.

Nutritional Analysis: Quantity of Energy in Calories: 50, Quantity of Fat: 4g, Quantity of Protein: 2g, Carbs: 4g, Quantity of Fiber: 2g

86. Lemon & Garlic Green Beans

Making and Duration Time: 7 minutes **Cooking Duration:** 12 minutes **Number of Portions:** 4
Required Material for this Recipe:
- Green legumes, freshly cut, 1 pound
- Minced garlic from two stems
- One tablespoon of olive oil
- Extract from one citrus
- Pepper and salt

Step By Step Instructions for Recipe:
1. Put the green beans in a saucepan of seasoned water and bring it to a boil.
2. Put in the oven for 3–4 minutes.
3. The legumes, once drained, should be cooked with olive oil and chopped garlic.
4. To taste the garlic, cook it for 3–4 minutes over medium heat.
5. Turn off the stove and squeeze in some lemon.
6. Add salt and pepper to taste, then serve.

Nutritional Analysis: Quantity of Energy in Calories: 50, Quantity of Fat: 3g, Quantity of Protein: 2g, Carbs: 6g, Quantity of Fiber: 4g

87. Sweet Potato Wedges

Making and Duration Time: 5 minutes **Cooking Duration:** 25 minutes **Number of Portions:** 4

Required Material for this Recipe:
- Two sweet potatoes, average in size, sliced into slices.
- One tablespoon of olive oil

- An ounce of pepper
- Pepper and salt

Step By Step Instructions for Recipe:
1. Turn the oven on to 400 degrees.
2. Prepare an oven tray by spreading sweet potato slices in a single row.
3. Olive oil and smoky paprika are great additions.
4. Sprinkle some salt and pepper on it.
5. Serve after 20–25 minutes of roasting.

Nutritional Analysis: Quantity of Energy in Calories: 90, Quantity of Fat: 3g, Quantity of Protein: 1g, Carbs: 15g, Quantity of Fiber: 3g

88. Garlic Roasted Broccoli

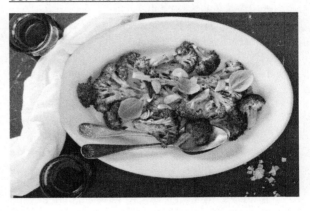

Making and Duration Time: 7 minutes **Cooking Duration:** 15 minutes **Number of Portions:** 4

Required Material for this Recipe:
- One stalk of broccoli, floriated.
- Olive oil, 2 tablespoons
- Three bulbs of garlic, chopped
- Half a teaspoon of pepper, a teaspoon of salt

Step By Step Instructions for Recipe:
1. Turn the oven on to 400 degrees.
2. Olive oil, garlic, salt, and pepper should be tossed with the broccoli stems.
3. Prepare a roasting tray with a single piece of broccoli.
4. Broccoli needs 15 minutes in the oven to become soft and caramelized. Serve

Nutritional Analysis: Quantity of Energy in Calories: 83, Quantity of Carbs: 7g, Quantity of Protein: 3g, Quantity of Fat: 6g, Quantity of Fiber: 3g.

89. Quinoa Salad

Making and Duration Time: 10 minutes **Cooking Duration:** 20 minutes **Number of Portions:** 4

Required Material for this Recipe:
- About a cup of quinoa
- The equivalent of two glasses of water
- One-fourth cup of red onion, chopped
- One-half cup of each chopped cucumber, sliced cherry tomatoes
- Fresh parsley, minced; one-fourth cup
- Lemon juice, 2 tablespoons
- Olive oil, 2 tablespoons
- half teaspoon Salt
- a pinch of pepper, roughly a quarter of a teaspoon

Step By Step Instructions for Recipe:
1. Drain the quinoa thoroughly after washing it in a fine-mesh strainer.
2. Cook the quinoa in a pot of boiling water.
3. Turn the heat down to low, cover the saucepan, and let the quinoa cook until soft, and the water is absorbed, about 15 to 20 minutes.
4. Transfer it to a big dish.
5. Toss together the red onion, cucumber, cherry tomatoes, olive oil, parsley, salt, and pepper. Serve

Nutritional Analysis: Quantity of Energy in Calories: 194, Quantity of Carbs: 26g, Quantity of Protein: 6g, Quantity of Fat: 8g, Quantity of Fiber: 4g

90. Roasted Asparagus with Parmesan Cheese and Lemon

Making and Duration Time: 6 minutes **Cooking Duration:** 10 minutes **Number of Portions:** 4

Required Material for this Recipe:
- 1 pound of asparagus, cut off the tips
- 2 tablespoons olive oil
- Two finely chopped garlic cloves
- A pinch of salt
- A Pinch of Pepper
- One-fourth cup of shredded Parmesan
- Lemon juice, 1 tablespoon

Step By Step Instructions for Recipe:
1. Prepare a 425°F oven.
2. Mix the asparagus with the garlic, olive oil, salt, and pepper in a dish.
3. Put the asparagus on a baking tray in a single row. Asparagus needs to be cooked for 10 minutes to become delicate and caramelized.
4. Sprinkle with Parmesan and squeeze fresh lemon over the hot dish. Serve

Nutritional Analysis: Quantity of Energy in Calories: 89, Quantity of Carbs: 5g, Quantity of Protein: 5g, Quantity of Fat: 7g, Quantity of Fiber: 2g

91. Lemon and Garlic Toasted Asparagus

Making and Duration Time: 7 minutes **Cooking Duration:** 10 minutes **Number of Portions:** 4

Required Material for this Recipe:
- Asparagus, weighing one pound
- Olive oil, enough for 2 teaspoons
- Two hands full of chopped garlic
- Juice and rind from a single lemon.
- Pepper and salt

Step By Step Instructions for Recipe:
1. Preheat the cooking temperature to 425 degrees.
2. Once the asparagus has been cleaned, cut off the spiny ends. Olive oil, garlic, fresh lemon juice, and lemon flavor should all be mixed together.
3. Spread the asparagus out on a baking sheet and pour the oil combination over them.
4. Put in some pepper and salt.
5. Brown and soften in the oven for 10 minutes. Keep warm

Nutritional Analysis: Quantity of Energy in Calories: 84, Quantity of Fat: 7g, Quantity of Protein: 2g, Quantity of Carbs: 5g, Quantity of Fiber: 2g

92. Grilled Zucchini with Mint and Lemon

Making and Duration Time: 5 minutes **Cooking Duration:** 8 minutes **Number of Portions:** 4

Required Material for this Recipe:
- Thinly slice 2 medium-sized zucchinis
- 1 ounce of olive oil

- One lemon, squeezed and rind removed
- 1 cup of fresh mint leaves, minced
- Pepper and salt

Step By Step Instructions for Recipe:
1. Prepare a medium fire in the griddle.
2. Olive oil, lemon juice, lemon peel, and herbs should be whisked together.
3. Coat the zucchini rounds with the olive oil concoction. Put in some pepper and salt.
4. To broil the zucchini and achieve grill lines and tenderness, place the segments on the griddle and roast for 4 minutes on each side. Keep warm.

Nutritional Analysis: Quantity of Energy in Calories: 59, Quantity of Fat: 5g, Quantity of Protein: 1g, Quantity of Carbs: 4g, Quantity of Fiber: 1g

93. Roasted Brussels Sprouts with Balsamic Glaze

Making and Duration Time: 6 minutes **Cooking Duration:** 20 minutes **Number of Portions:** 4

Required Material for this Recipe:
- Divided Brussels stems weighing 1 pound
- Olive oil, enough for 2 teaspoons
- Pepper and salt
- Mix together 2 tbsp. balsamic vinegar and 1 tbsp. honey.

Step By Step Instructions for Recipe:
1. Preheat the oven to 425 degrees.
2. Combine the Brussels sprouts, olive oil, salt, and pepper in a dish and toss.
3. The Brussels sprouts should be roasted for 15 to 20 minutes, or until soft and beginning to brown, depending on how large they are.
4. Over medium heat, whisk together balsamic vinegar and honey for 5 minutes, or until the liquid solidifies.
5. Serve the broiled Brussels sprouts immediately with the balsamic sauce.

Nutritional Analysis: Quantity of Energy in Calories: 123, Quantity of Fat: 8g, Quantity of Protein: 3g, Quantity of Carbs: 14g, Quantity of Fiber: 4g

94. Lemon Garlic Broccolini

Making and Duration Time: 7 minutes **Cooking Duration:** 13 minutes **Number of Portions:** 4

Required Material for this Recipe:
- Broccoli, one pound
- Olive oil, enough for 2 teaspoons
- Four garlic bulbs, chopped
- Zested and juiced lemon, 1
- Pepper and salt

Step By Step Instructions for Recipe:
1. Chop the broccolini into small pieces after trimming the edges.
2. In a pan, warm the olive oil over medium heat.
3. Add the garlic and simmer for 1–2 minutes, or until the garlic smell is mellow.
4. Sauté the broccolini in the garlic oil for 5–7 minutes, occasionally stirring, until tender.
5. Turn off the stove and stir in the lemon peel and juice. Add salt and pepper to taste and serve immediately.

Nutritional Analysis: Quantity of Energy in Calories: 87, Quantity of Fat: 7g, Quantity of Protein: 2g, Quantity of Carbs: 5g, Quantity of Fiber: 2g

95. Garlic Sautéed Carrots

Making and Duration Time: 6 minutes **Cooking Duration:** 25 minutes **Number of Portions:** 4

Required Material for this Recipe:
- Baby carrots, one pound, cleaned and desiccated
- Olive oil, enough for two teaspoons
- Four garlic bulbs, chopped
- Pepper and salt

Step By Step Instructions for Recipe:
1. Turn the oven on to 400 degrees.
2. Using a mixing bowl, toss together the baby carrots, olive oil, garlic, salt, and pepper.
3. Spread the carrots out on a baking sheet and broil them for 20 to 25 minutes, or until they are soft and starting to color. Serve.

Nutritional Analysis: Quantity of Energy in Calories: 87, Quantity of Fat: 7g, Quantity of Protein: 1g, Quantity of Carbs: 7g, Quantity of Fiber: 2g

96. Lemon Herb Quinoa with Mint

Making and Duration Time: 5 minutes **Cooking Duration:** 20 minutes **Number of Portions:** 4

Required Material for this Recipe:
- One serving (or one cup) of quinoa
- The equivalent of two glasses of water
- Olive oil, enough for two teaspoons
- 1/4 cup of fresh lemon juice
- Finely chopped fresh cilantro, 2 tablespoons
- Mince two tablespoons of fresh mint.
- 1/4 teaspoons of salt
- 1/4 teaspoons of pepper

Step By Step Instructions for Recipe:
1. After washing the quinoa in a fine-mesh strainer, allow it to dry completely.
2. In a medium pot, bring the rice and water to a simmer.
3. Turn the heat down to low, cover the skillet, and let the quinoa boil for 15 to 20 minutes, or until soft.
4. Fluff the quinoa with a spatula and pour it into a large serving bowl.
5. Olive oil, lemon juice, cilantro, mint, salt, and pepper should all be added to the meal. Mix thoroughly and serve.

Nutritional Analysis: Quantity of Energy in Calories: 200, Quantity of Fat: 8g, Quantity of Protein: 6g, Quantity of Carbs: 27g, Quantity of Fiber: 3g

97. Spicy Grilled Carrots

Making and Duration Time: 8 minutes **Cooking Duration:** 25 minutes **Number of Portions:** 4

Required Material for this Recipe:
- Carrots, trimmed and cut, 1 pound
- Olive oil, 2 tablespoons
- 1/2 teaspoons of cumin
- 1/2 teaspoons of smoky paprika
- A Pinch of Pepper
- 1/4 teaspoons of salt

Step By Step Instructions for Recipe:
1. Turn the oven on to 400 degrees.
2. Olive oil, cumin, smoky paprika, pepper, and salt should be tossed with the carrots.
3. Spread the carrots out in a single line on a baking tray.
4. For succulent, slightly caramelized results, roast in the oven for 25 minutes.

Nutritional Analysis: Quantity of Energy in Calories: 90, Quantity of Fat: 7g, Quantity of Protein: 1g, Quantity of Carbs: 7g, Quantity of Fiber: 2g

98. Mango & Avocado Salad

Making and Duration Time: 11 minutes **Number of Portions:** 4

Required Material for this Recipe:
- Two mangos skinned and sliced.
- You'll need two avocados, cleaned and sliced.
- One-fourth cup of minced red onion
- One lime's worth of juice
- Two tablespoons of minced parsley
- Pepper and salt

Step By Step Instructions for Recipe:
1. Mango, avocado, red onion, parsley, lime juice, salt, and pepper should all be combined.
2. Mix thoroughly by tossing.
3. Immediately serve.

Nutritional Analysis: Quantity of Energy in Calories: 213, Quantity of Fat: 14g, Quantity of Carbs: 24g, Quantity of Fiber: 8g, Quantity of Protein: 3g

99. Roasted Turmeric Cabbage

Making and Duration Time: 10 minutes **Cooking Duration:** 25 minutes **Number of Portions:** 4

Required Material for this Recipe:
- Cut flowers from a cabbage
- Olive oil, enough for two teaspoons
- Turmeric, about one spoonful
- a pinch of dried garlic
- Paprika, 1/2 tsp
- Pepper and salt

Step By Step Instructions for Recipe:

1. Preheat the oven to 425 degrees.
2. Olive oil, turmeric, garlic powder, paprika, salt, and pepper should be used to cover cabbage pieces before they are tossed in a bowl and cooked.
3. Spread the cabbage out in a single line on a baking tray.
4. Cook in the oven for 20–25 minutes, or until soft and just beginning to color. Keep warm.

Nutritional Analysis: Quantity of Energy in Calories: 93 kcal, Quantity of Fat: 7 g, Quantity of Protein: 4 g, Quantity of Carbs: 8 g, Quantity of Fiber: 3 g

CHAPTER 7: SNACKS AND DESSERT RECIPE

99. Chocolate Avocado Pudding

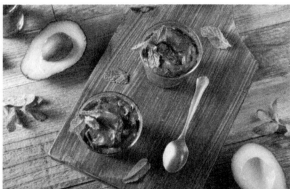

Making and Duration Time: 13 minutes
Number of Portions: 2

Required Material for this Recipe:
- A single mature avocado
- Singular Ripe Banana
- Sugar-free chocolate powder, 2 tablespoons
- The equivalent of two tablespoons of maple sugar
- An Extract of Vanilla, 1/4 Teaspoon
- 1/2 teaspoon of almond extract

Step By Step Instructions for Recipe:
1. Blend all the components together until they are completely combined.
2. Split it between two individual containers and chill for 30 minutes. Serve.

Nutritional Analysis: Quantity of Energy in Calories: 217, Quantity of Fat: 12g, Quantity of Protein: 4g, Quantity of Carbs: 31g, Quantity of Fiber: 7g

100. Turmeric Grilled Chick Peas

Making and Duration Time: 7 minutes **Cooking Duration:** 25 minutes **Number of Portions:** 4

Required Material for this Recipe:
- A can of chickpeas that has been emptied and washed

- An olive oil pinch
- One-half teaspoon of turmeric powder
- Smoked paprika, 1/2 teaspoon
- Powdered garlic, half a teaspoon
- Pepper and salt

Step By Step Instructions for Recipe:
1. Turn the oven on to 400 degrees.
2. Olive oil, turmeric, smoky paprika, garlic powder, salt, and pepper should be used to cover the legumes.
3. Place the legumes in a single line on a cookie tray.
4. Crisp up in the oven for 20 to 25 minutes.
5. Take it out of the oven, let it chill, serve.

Nutritional Analysis: Quantity of Energy in Calories: 102, Quantity of Fat: 3g, Quantity of Protein: 4g, Quantity of Carbs: 16g, Quantity of Fiber: 4g

101. Banana Oatmeal Cookies

Making and Duration Time: 10 minutes **Cooking Duration:** 15 minutes **Number of Portions:** 12

Required Material for this Recipe:
- Two mature bananas, pureed.
- Almond butter. 1-quarter cup, 1/2 cup dry oats
- One-fourth cup of maple sugar
- Applesauce, 1/4 cup, sugar-free
- One vanilla essence teaspoon
- One-half teaspoon of cinnamon powder
- 1/4 teaspoons of salt

Step By Step Instructions for Recipe:
1. Prepare a 350°F oven.
2. Mix everything together in a large bowl.
3. Make little peaks with a spoon and set them on a baking sheet lined with parchment paper.
4. Flatten each biscuit slightly with the back of the spatula.

5. Golden brown, about 15 minutes in the oven.
6. Remove from oven, set aside to chill, and then serve.

Nutritional information: Quantity of Energy in Calories: 97, Quantity of Fat: 3g, Quantity of Protein: 3g, Quantity of Carbs: 16g, Quantity of Fiber: 2g

102. Chocolate Banana Bites

Making and Duration Time: 12 minutes
Number of Portions: 4

Required Material for this Recipe:
- Fruits: 2 big bananas
- One-fourth cup of semisweet chocolate chunks
- One-fourth cup of minced walnuts
- A little salt

Step By Step Instructions for Recipe:
1. Bananas should be peeled and chopped into bite-sized chunks.
2. To warm the chocolate, you can either use a microwave or a double pot.
3. Half-submerge the banana pieces in the melted chocolate and set them on a parchment-lined baking sheet.
4. Chop some walnuts and sprinkle some salt on top of the chocolate-covered banana segments.
5. Put them in the fridge for ten minutes, or until the chocolate has hardened.

Nutritional Analysis: Quantity of Energy in Calories: 112, Quantity of Fat: 6g, Quantity of Carbs: 17g, Quantity of Fiber: 3g, Quantity of Protein: 2g

103. Peanut Butter Protein Balls

Making and Duration Time: 11 minutes
Number of Portions: 8

Required Material for this Recipe:
- Roughly one cup of grains
- One-half cup of peanut butter
- 1/2 tsp. of butter
- Shredded coconut, sugar-free, 1/4 cup
- Flaxseed meal, about a quarter cup

- One-fourth cup of semisweet chocolate chunks

Step By Step Instructions for Recipe:
1. Toss together all of the seasonings.
2. Form the dough into eight spheres of uniform dimension.
3. Put in the fridge for at least 30 minutes before serving.

Nutritional Analysis: Quantity of Energy in Calories: 238, Quantity of Fat: 13g, Quantity of Carbs: 24g, Quantity of Fiber: 4g, Quantity of Protein: 8g

104. Mango Chia Pudding

Making and Duration Time: 8 minutes **Number of Portions:** 2

Required Material for this Recipe:
- 1 mature mango, skinned and chopped
- Almond milk, sweetener-free, 1 cup
- A quarter cup of chia seeds
- An Extract of Vanilla, 1/4 Teaspoon
- 1 tsp honey (optional)

Step By Step Instructions for Recipe:
1. Mix the coconut milk with the diced mango in a blender until homogeneous.
2. Combine the blended mango and almond milk, chia seeds, vanilla essence, and honey (if using) in a mixing bowl.
3. After 5 minutes, give it another toss to break up any clumps that may have formed.
4. Put in the fridge for 30 minutes, or until the pudding has thickened.

Nutritional Analysis: Quantity of Energy in Calories: 216, Quantity of Fat: 11g, Quantity of Carbs: 28g, Quantity of Fiber: 12g, Quantity of Protein: 7g

105. Chocolate Berry Smoothie Bowl

Making and Duration Time: 6 minutes **Number of Portions:** 1

Required Material for this Recipe:
- One frozen banana
- Half a cup of frozen mixed berries and half a cup of almond milk
- A spoonful of cocoa powder

- The same proportion of 1/2 teaspoon of powdered cinnamon, vanilla essence
- Any toppings you like (fresh berries, sliced banana, coconut flakes, minced almonds, etc.)

Step By Step Instructions for Recipe:
1. To make a delicious smoothie, combine frozen bananas, assorted fruit, almond milk, cocoa powder, cinnamon, and vanilla essence in a blender and process until creamy.
2. Place the blended drink in a serving dish and top it with the topping of your choice.

Nutritional Analysis: Quantity of Energy in Calories: 235, Quantity of Protein: 4g, Quantity of Fat: 6g, Quantity of Carbs: 46g, Quantity of Fiber: 8g

106. Baked Apple Chips

Making and Duration Time: 7 minutes **Cooking Duration:** 1-hour **Number of Portions:** 2

Required Material for this Recipe:
- Two peeled and finely cut apples
- Two teaspoons of honey
- Ground cinnamon, one teaspoon

Step By Step Instructions for Recipe:
1. Turn the oven on to 400 degrees.
2. Upon a baking tray, spread out some parchment paper.
3. Spread the honey and cinnamon over the apple segments and stir to moisten.
4. Spread the apple pieces out in a single line on the baking tray.
5. Prepare until crunchy and golden, 45-60 minutes, turning the pieces over once.
6. Wait a few minutes for the apple crisps to settle, and then serve.

Nutritional Analysis: Quantity of Energy in Calories: 102, Quantity of Protein: 0g, Quantity of Fat: 0g, Quantity of Carbs: 27g, Quantity of Fiber: 4g

107. Chocolate Peanut Butter Energy Bites

Making and Duration Time: 11 minutes **Number of Portions:** 12

Required Material for this Recipe:
- Roughly one cup of oats

- One-fourth cup of smooth peanut butter
- 1-fourth of a cup of honey
- 1/2 teaspoon pulverized chia seeds
- chocolate powder, sugar-free, 1/4 cup
- 1- quarter cup chocolate chips

Step By Step Instructions for Recipe:
1. Toss all the ingredients together in a dish.
2. Form the dough into 12 equal-sized spheres using your palms.
3. Place the energy morsels on a platter and place it in the refrigerator for 30 minutes to harden.

Nutritional Analysis: Quantity of Energy in Calories: 130, Quantity of Protein: 4g, Quantity of Fat: 7g, Quantity of Carbs: 15g, Quantity of Fiber: 3g

108. Chocolate Almond Butter Cups

Making and Duration Time: 10 minutes **Number of Portions:** 8

Required Material for this Recipe:
- One-half cup of almond butter
- Coconut oil, softened, about a quarter cup
- Powdered raw cocoa, one-fourth cup
- Maple syrup, 2 tablespoons
- Vanilla essence, 1/2 teaspoon
- A little salt

Step By Step Instructions for Recipe:
1. Blend together the almond butter, warmed coconut oil, cocoa powder, maple syrup, vanilla essence, and a sprinkle of salt.
2. Muffin tins can be lined with silicone liners or paper plates.
3. Divide the chocolate mixture in half and pour half into each cup.
4. Wait 5-10 minutes for the muffins to solidify in the fridge.
5. When the chocolate has set, apply a thin coating of almond butter over each layer and top with the remaining chocolate. Refreeze the muffin pan for 5-10 minutes to ensure a firm result.
6. Assemble cold

Nutritional Analysis: Quantity of Energy in Calories: 182kcal | Quantity of Fat: 17g | Quantity of Carbs: 7g | Quantity of Fiber: 3g | Quantity of Protein: 4

109. Baked Pear Chips

Making and Duration Time: 12 minutes **Cooking Duration:** 2- hours **Number of Portions:** 4

Required Material for this Recipe:
- Two pears, cut very thickly
- A pinch of spice
- Two tablespoons of honey
- A little salt

Step By Step Instructions for Recipe:
1. Prepare a 200-degree oven.
2. Upon a baking tray, spread out some parchment paper.
3. Mix the honey, cinnamon, and salt in a bowl, then add the apple segments and toss to moisten.
4. Prepare a baking tray by laying out a single layer of apple segments.
5. Apple segments should be baked for two hours to achieve a buttery crunchy texture.
6. Allow them to chill completely before serving.

Nutritional Analysis: Quantity of Energy in Calories: 69kcal, Quantity of Fat: 0.3g, Quantity of Carbs: 18g, Quantity of Fiber: 3g, Quantity of Protein: 0.3g

110. Peanut Butter Banana Ice Cream

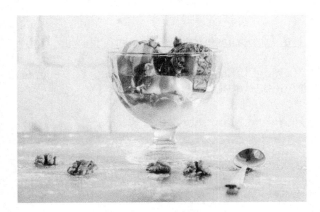

Making and Duration Time: 6 minutes **Number of Portions:** 2

Required Material for this Recipe:
- 2 mature bananas, cut, and refrigerated
- Creamy peanut butter, 2 tablespoons
- An Extract of Vanilla, 1/4 Teaspoon

- A little salt

Step By Step Instructions for Recipe:
1. peanut butter, vanilla essence, salt, and frozen banana segments should be blended in a high-speed mixer, to obtain a creamy and smooth mix.
2. You can eat it right away, or you can put it in a jar and refrigerate it.

Nutritional Analysis: Quantity of Energy in Calories: 168kcal, Quantity of Fat: 8g, Quantity of Carbs: 24g, Quantity of Fiber: 3g, Quantity of Protein: 6g

111. Chocolate Chia Pudding

Making and Duration Time: 7 minutes **Number of Portions:** 2

Required Material for this Recipe:
- 1/4 cup of chia seeds
- Almond milk, 1 cup, sugar-free
- 1/2 teaspoon of pure vanilla extract
- 2 tablespoons of cacao powder and maple syrup (1 of each)
- Extract Vanilla, Half a Teaspoon
- A little salt
- Nuts or berries (extra)

Step By Step Instructions for Recipe:
1. Put the chia seeds in a dish and add the almond milk, cocoa powder, maple syrup, vanilla essence, and salt.
2. Put it in the freezer for at least two hours or overnight, and make sure it's covered.
3. At serving time, give it a good mix and then garnish it with whatever fruit or nuts you like.

Nutritional Analysis: Quantity of Energy in Calories: 160, Quantity of Protein: 4g, Quantity of Fat: 9g, Carbs: 17g, Quantity of Fiber: 11g

112. Roasted Cinnamon Potato Bites

Making and Duration Time: 12 minutes **Cooking Duration:** 25 minutes **Number of Portions:** 4

Required Material for this Recipe:
- Two medium-sized potatoes cleaned and diced.
- Coconut oil, softened, a teaspoonful

- Cinnamon, one tablespoon's worth
- 1/2 milligram of salt

Step By Step Instructions for Recipe:
1. Turn the oven on to 400 degrees.
2. Mix the cinnamon, salt, heated coconut oil, and diced sweet potatoes together.
3. Spread the mixture out on a baking sheet and broil it for 25 minutes, or until it is soft and just beginning to color. Serve

Nutritional Analysis: Quantity of Energy in Calories: 90, Quantity of Protein: 1g, Quantity of Fat: 3g, Carbs: 16g, Quantity of Fiber: 3g

113. Berry Yogurt

Making and Duration Time: 4 minutes **Number of Portions:** 1

Required Material for this Recipe:
- One-half cup of unsweetened Greek yogurt
- Mixed fruit, half a cup
- One-fourth cup of cereal
- 1.5 grams of honey

Step By Step Instructions for Recipe:
1. Greek yogurt, cereal, and assorted fruit go in a container in that order.
2. Add some honey for flavor.
3. Assemble cold

Nutritional Analysis: Quantity of Energy in Calories: 270, Quantity of Protein: 17g, Quantity of Fat: 6g, Carbs: 44g, Quantity of Fiber: 6g

114. Spiced Roasted Nuts

Making and Duration Time: 4 minutes **Cooking Duration:** 12 minutes **Number of Portions:** 6

Required Material for this Recipe:
- Two tablespoons of uncooked nuts assortment (almonds, cashews, pecans)
- An ounce and a half of coconut oil
- One teaspoon of cinnamon powder
- 1/2 teaspoon of ginger powder
- A pinch of salt

Step By Step Instructions for Recipe:
1. Prepare a 350°F oven.
2. Combine the almonds with coconut oil, spices, and seasonings.

3. Spread the nuts out on a baking sheet coated with parchment paper.
4. Stir midway through roasting time to ensure even browning.
5. Allow the almonds to settle to room temperature before serving.

Nutritional Analysis: Quantity of Energy in Calories: 240, Quantity of Protein: 6g, Quantity of Fat: 21g, Quantity of Carbs: 10g, Quantity of Fiber: 3g

115. Strawberry Banana Smoothie

Making and Duration Time: 5 minutes **Number of Portions:** 1

Required Material for this Recipe:
- Singular Ripe Banana
- Frozen blackberries, one cup
- Almond milk, sugar-free, 1/2 cup
- Mix in 1/2 teaspoon of honey.
- Cinnamon, powdered, 1/4 teaspoon

Step By Step Instructions for Recipe:
1. Put everything in a blender and blend until it's smooth.
2. The drink can be served immediately after being poured into a glass.

Nutritional Analysis: Quantity of Energy in Calories: 174, Quantity of Protein: 3g, Quantity of Fat: 3g, Quantity of Carbs: 37g, Quantity of Fiber: 7g

116. Chocolate Peanut Butter Energy Balls

Making and Duration Time: 11 minutes **Number of Portions:** 12 balls

Required Material for this Recipe:
- Oatmeal rolled: 1 cup
- Natural peanut butter, half a cup
- 1/2 tsp. of butter
- Sugar-free chocolate powder, about a quarter cup
- Vanilla essence, 1 teaspoon
- 1/4 teaspoon of salt

Step By Step Instructions for Recipe:
1. Combine all of the components by stirring them together.
2. Form the mixture into 1-inch rounds using a cookie spatula or a utensil.

3. Chill the spheres in the refrigerator for at least 30 minutes before serving.

Nutrition information (per ball): Quantity of Energy in Calories: 125, Quantity of Fat: 6g, Quantity of Carbs: 15g, Quantity of Protein: 4g, Quantity of Fiber: 2g

117. Mango Salsa

Making and Duration Time: 10 minutes **Cooking Duration:** 0 minutes **Number of Portions:** 4

Required Material for this Recipe:
- 2 mature mangoes, sliced
- One scarlet bell pepper, sliced
- Half an onion, sliced scarlet
- 1/4 cup of cilantro, minced
- 1/2 teaspoon of salt 1 squeezed lime

Step By Step Instructions for Recipe:
1. Combine everything by stirring it together.
2. Refrigerate until ready to serve or serve right away.

Nutrition information: Quantity of Energy in Calories: 70, Quantity of Fat: 0g, Quantity of Carbs: 18g, Quantity of Protein: 1g, Quantity of Fiber: 2g

118. Blueberry Oat Bars

Making and Duration Time: 8 minutes **Cooking Duration:** 20 minutes **Number of Portions:** 8 bars

Required Material for this Recipe:
- Roll your own two cups of oats
- 1/4 cup peanut butter
- About a third of a cup of honey
- 1/4 cup unsweetened apple juice
- 1/2 tsp almond extract
- 1/2 teaspoons of cinnamon powder
- Half a teaspoon of salt One cup of blackberries

Step By Step Instructions for Recipe:
1. Preheat oven to 350 degrees Fahrenheit and line an 8x8-inch baking dish with parchment paper. Mix all ingredients except blueberries and stir well. Fold in blueberries.
2. Bake for 20-25 minutes, or until the edges are beginning to brown.

3. Let cool before cutting into 8 bars.

Nutrition information (per bar): Quantity of Energy in Calories: 256, Quantity of Fat: 10g, Quantity of Carbs: 36g, Quantity of Protein: 7g, Quantity of Fiber: 4g

119. Roasted Turmeric Chick Peas

Making and Duration Time: 5 minutes **Cooking Duration:** 30 minutes **Number of Portions:** 4

Required Material for this Recipe:
- Two cans of legumes (chickpeas), drained and washed
- Two teaspoons of butter
- Turmeric, about one spoonful
- A pinch of coriander
- a pinch of dried garlic
- Salt one-fourth of a spoonful

Step By Step Instructions for Recipe:
1. Turn the oven on to 400 degrees.
2. On a baking sheet lined with parchment paper, disperse the legumes.
3. Toss the beans with olive oil to moisten them. Add the salt, turmeric, coriander, and garlic powder to the beans and stir to combine. Mix by tossing.
4. After 30 minutes in the oven, flipping once or twice, the food should be crunchy and golden brown. Serve.

Nutritional Analysis: Quantity of Energy in Calories: 193, Quantity of Fat: 6g, Quantity of Protein: 8g, Quantity of Carbs: 29g, Quantity of Fiber: 8g

120. Peanut Butter and Banana Bites

Making and Duration Time: 7 minutes **Cooking Duration:** 0 minutes **Number of Portions:** 2

Required Material for this Recipe:
- Sliced circles of a single banana
- Add 2 tbsp. of peanut butter.
- Chia nuts, one teaspoonful
- 1 tbsp grated coconut, sugar-free

Step By Step Instructions for Recipe:
1. Cover each banana piece with peanut butter.
2. Top the peanut butter with chia seeds and coconut flakes. Serve

Nutritional information: Quantity of Energy in Calories: 198, Quantity of Fat: 11g, Quantity of Protein: 6g, Quantity of Carbs: 23g, Quantity of Fiber: 6g

121. Roasted Potato Chips

Making and Duration Time: 13 minutes **Cooking Duration:** 25 minutes **Number of Portions:** 4

Required Material for this Recipe:
- Two large potatoes sliced paper-thin.
- Olive oil, 2 tablespoons
- A pinch of salt
- 1/4 teaspoon of onion powder
- A Pinch of Pepper

Step By Step Instructions for Recipe:
1. Turn the oven on to 400 degrees.
2. Oil, salt, garlic powder, and black pepper should be used to cover the sweet potato pieces in a dish.
3. Spread the potato pieces out in a single line on a baking tray.
4. Crisp up in the oven at a high temperature for 20–25 minutes, rotating once.
5. Remove from oven and allow to cool slightly before serving.

Nutritional Analysis: Quantity of Energy in Calories: 146, Quantity of Fat: 7.6g, Quantity of Carbs: 19.8g, Quantity of Fiber: 3.5g, Quantity of Protein: 1.8g

122. Greek Yogurt with Berries and Almonds

Making and Duration Time: 6 minutes **Number of Portions:** 1

Required Material for this Recipe:
- One-half cup of unsweetened Greek yogurt
- Mixed cherries, 1/4 cup (such as blueberries, raspberries, and strawberries)
- One Tablespoon of Almonds, Sliced
- Honey, half a spoonful

Step By Step Instructions for Recipe:
1. Mix honey into Greek yogurt.
2. Add chopped almonds and a mixture of fruit for garnish.
3. Immediately serve.

Nutritional Analysis: Quantity of Energy in Calories: 140, Quantity of Fat: 5g, Quantity of Carbs: 12g, Quantity of Fiber: 2g, Quantity of Protein: 13g

123. Baked Cinnamon Apples

Making and Duration Time: 11 minutes **Cooking Duration:** 30 minutes **Number of Portions:** 4

Required Material for this Recipe:
- Core and thinly slice 4 medium-sized Apples.
- Add 2 tbsp. of maple syrup.
- An ounce and a half of coconut oil
- Ground cinnamon, one teaspoon
- 1/4 tablespoon of ginger powder
- Ground Nutmeg, 1/4 Teaspoon
- A little salt

Step By Step Instructions for Recipe:
1. Preheat the oven to 375 degrees.
2. Mix the maple syrup, coconut oil, cinnamon, ginger, nutmeg, and salt together in a bowl, then add the apple segments and toss to moisten.
3. Spread the apple concoction in a casserole dish with a spoon.
4. Apples should be browned and soft after 25-30 minutes in the oven.
5. If preferred, top with a spoonful of coconut cream or some minced almonds and serve heatedly.

Nutritional Analysis: Quantity of Energy in Calories: 134 kcal, Quantity of Fat: 3 g, Quantity of Protein: 0 g, Quantity of Carbs: 30 g, Quantity of Fiber: 5 g

CHAPTER 8: BREAD RECIPES

124. Almond Flour Banana Loaf

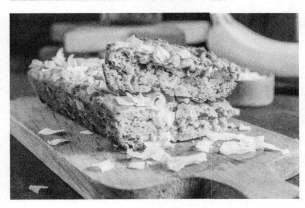

Making and Duration Time: 10 minutes **Cooking Duration:** 45 minutes **Number of Portions:** 8

Required Material for this Recipe:
- Three mature bananas, pureed.
- 3 eggs
- Maple syrup, 1-quarter mug
- Coconut oil, warmed, 1/4 cup
- 1/2 tsp vanilla extract
- Almond flour, two tablespoons
- 1 teaspoon of baking powder plus 1/2 baking soda
- Cinnamon, 1/2 teaspoon
- 1/4 teaspoons of salt

Step By Step Instructions for Recipe:
1. Prepare a 350°F oven. Grease a 9-by-5-inch bread pan.
2. Combine the pureed bananas, eggs, maple syrup, coconut oil, and vanilla essence in a dish.
3. In a separate dish, combine the baking powder, salt, almond flour, baking soda, and cinnamon.
4. It's time to blend the dry and liquid components.
5. Fill the prepped bread container with the mixture.

6. A skewer put into the middle of the Loaf should come out clear after 40 to 45 minutes of baking time.
7. After ten minutes, remove the bread from the skillet and place it on a metal rack to chill completely.

Nutritional Analysis: Quantity of Energy in Calories: 297, Quantity of Fat: 22g, Quantity of Carbs: 19g, Quantity of Fiber: 4g, Quantity of Protein: 8g

125. Zucchini Loaf

Making and Duration Time: 15 minutes **Cooking Duration:** 50 minutes **Number of Portions:** 8

Required Material for this Recipe:
- Almond flour: 1 1/2 teaspoons
- One-half cup of coconut flour
- Just a pinch of baking powder
- 1/4 teaspoon of baking soda
- Cinnamon, 1/2 teaspoon
- 3 eggs, 1/4 teaspoon of salt
- 1/2 tsp. maple syrup
- Coconut oil, warmed, 1/4 cup
- One vanilla essence teaspoon
- Zucchini, shredded, one cup (1 medium zucchini)
- Walnuts, 1-quarter cup

Step By Step Instructions for Recipe:
1. Prepare a 350°F oven. Grease a 9-by-5-inch bread pan.
2. Put together some flour (almond, coconut, baking soda, baking powder, cinnamon, and salt) in a dish.
3. In another dish, beat together eggs, maple syrup, heated coconut oil, and vanilla essence.
4. Remember to add the chopped zucchini.
5. After incorporating the liquid ingredients, mix them in completely with the dry ones.
6. Add the ground walnuts, too.

7. Pour the mixture into the prepped bread pan.
8. Wait 45-50 minutes, or until a skewer placed in the center comes out clean, before taking the loaf out of the oven.
9. After ten minutes, remove the bread from the skillet and place it on a metal rack to chill completely.

Nutritional Analysis: Quantity of Energy in Calories: 267, Quantity of Fat: 18g, Quantity of Carbs: 19g, Quantity of Fiber: 6g, Quantity of Protein: 9g

126. Paleo Pumpkin Loaf

Making and Duration Time: 12 minutes **Cooking Duration:** 50 minutes **Number of Portions:** 10

Required Material for this Recipe:
- Almond meal equaling one cup
- One-half cup of coconut flour
- one teaspoon of each baking powder, and baking soda
- a pinch of cinnamon
- 1/2 teaspoon of ginger powder
- one-fourth of a teaspoon of nutmeg
- a pinch of salt, four eggs
- Pumpkin purée, 1/2 cup
- 1/2 tsp. honey
- Coconut oil, warmed, 1/4 cup
- A splash of vanilla essence

Step By Step Instructions for Recipe:
1. Prepare a 350°F oven. Grease a 9-by-5-inch bread pan.
2. Combine the coconut flour, almond flour, baking powder, soda, and spices (cinnamon, ginger, nutmeg, and salt) in a dish.
3. In a separate dish, combine the heated coconut oil with the honey, eggs, pumpkin purée, and vanilla essence.
4. Add the liquid components to the dry ones, then mix everything together.
5. To the ready bread plate, add the mixture.
6. Keep cooking until a skewer put in the center comes out clean, about 40 to 50 minutes.
7. After ten minutes, remove the bread from the skillet.

8. Place it on a metal rack to chill completely.

Nutritional Analysis: Quantity of Energy in Calories: 161, Quantity of Fat: 10g, Quantity of Carbs: 13g, Quantity of Fiber: 5g, Quantity of Protein: 6g

127. Carrots & Zucchini Loaf

Making and Duration Time: 15 minutes **Cooking Duration:** 50 minutes **Number of Portions:** 10

Required Material for this Recipe:
- Almond flour measuring a cup
- One-half cup of coconut flour
- Baking soda, one teaspoon
- Baking powder, 1/2 teaspoon
- 1/4 tsp of cinnamon
- A pinch of nutmeg, about a quarter teaspoon
- 1/4 teaspoon of salt
- 4 eggs
- One-half cup of shredded carrots (1 medium carrot)
- sliced zucchini equaling 1/2 cup (1 medium zucchini)
- 1/2 tsp. honey
- Coconut oil, warmed, 1/4 cup
- A splash of vanilla essence

Step By Step Instructions for Recipe:
1. Prepare a 350°F oven. Grease a 9-by-5-inch bread pan.
2. To make the batter, combine the coconut flour, almond flour, baking powder, baking soda, cinnamon, nutmeg, and salt in a dish.
3. In another dish, whisk together eggs, carrots, zucchini, honey, heated coconut oil, and vanilla essence.
4. Add the liquid components to the dry ones, then mix everything together.
5. To the ready bread plate, add the mixture.
6. Keep cooking until a skewer put in the center comes out clean, 40 to 50 minutes.
7. After ten minutes, remove the bread from the skillet and place it on a metal rack to chill completely.

Nutritional Analysis: Quantity of Energy in Calories: 161, Quantity of Fat: 10g, Quantity of Carbs: 12g, Quantity of Fiber: 5g, Quantity of Protein: 6g

128. Savory Rosemary Almond Flour Bread

Making and Duration Time: 13 minutes **Cooking Duration:** 45 minutes **Number of Portions:** 8

Required Material for this Recipe:
- Almond flour, two tablespoons
- Arrowroot starch, 1/2 cup
- Just 1 tsp baking soda
- A pinch of salt
- Freshly cut rosemary, 1 tablespoon
- 3 eggs
- One-fourth cup of olive oil
- 1/4 cup of liquid (water)

Step By Step Instructions for Recipe:
1. Prepare a 350°F oven. Grease a bread pan that measures 8 by 4 inches.
2. Combine rosemary, arrowroot starch, baking soda, salt, and almond flour in a dish.
3. In a separate dish, combine the eggs, olive oil, and water.
4. Add the liquid components to the dry ones, then mix everything together.
5. To the ready bread plate, add the mixture.
6. Keep cooking until a skewer put in the center comes out clean, about 40 to 50 minutes.
7. After ten minutes, remove the bread from the skillet and place it on a metal rack to chill completely.

Nutritional Analysis: Quantity of Energy in Calories: 296, Quantity of Fat: 24g, Quantity of Carbs: 13g, Quantity of Fiber: 3g, Quantity of Protein: 9g

129. Sweet Potato & Banana Loaf

Making and Duration Time: 15 minutes **Cooking Duration:** 55 minutes **Number of Portions:** 12

Required Material for this Recipe:
- Almond flour, 1 1/2 teaspoons
- One-half cup of coconut flour
- Baking powder, one teaspoon
- Baking soda, half a teaspoon
- a pinch of spice, cinnamon
- one-fourth of a teaspoon of spice (nutmeg)
- A Pinch of Salt
- 3 eggs
- 1 roasted and pureed potato, medium (about 1 cup)
- Bananas, pureed, 2 mature
- 1/4 cup of coconut oil, heated
- One vanilla essence teaspoon

Step By Step Instructions for Recipe:
1. Prepare a 350°F oven. Grease a 9-by-5-inch bread pan.
2. To make the batter, combine the coconut flour, almond flour, baking powder, baking soda, cinnamon, nutmeg, and salt in a large dish.
3. In another dish, whisk together eggs, pureed sweet potato, crushed bananas, warmed coconut oil, and vanilla essence.
4. Add the liquid components to the dry ones, then mix everything together.
5. To the ready bread plate, add the mixture.
6. Keep cooking until a skewer put in the center comes out clean, about 40 to 50 minutes.
7. After ten minutes, remove the bread from the skillet and place it on a metal rack to chill completely.

Nutritional Analysis: Quantity of Energy in Calories: 187, Quantity of Fat: 11g, Quantity of Carbs: 17g, Quantity of Fiber: 5g, Quantity of Protein: 6g

130. Carrot Gingerbread

Making and Duration Time: 17 minutes **Cooking Duration:** 50 minutes **Number of Portions:** 12

Required Material for this Recipe:
- Almond flour, two tablespoons
- One-fourth cup of coconut flour
- Baking soda, one teaspoon
- Baking powder, 1/2 teaspoon
- A pinch of ginger powder
- One-half teaspoon of cinnamon powder
- 3 eggs, 1/4 teaspoon of salt
- 1/4 cup unsweetened apple juice
- 1/2 tsp. maple syrup
- Coconut oil, softened, about a quarter cup

- Grated carrots, one cup

Step By Step Instructions for Recipe:
1. Prepare a 350°F oven. Grease a 9-by-5-inch bread pan.
2. In a dish, combine the coconut flour, almond flour, baking powder, baking soda, ginger, cinnamon, and salt.
3. In a separate dish, combine the beaten eggs, applesauce, maple syrup, and heated coconut oil.
4. Add the liquid components to the dry ones, then mix everything together.
5. Add shredded carrots and mix well.
6. To the ready bread plate, add the mixture.
7. Keep cooking until a skewer put in the center comes out clean, about 40-50 minutes.
8. After ten minutes, remove the bread from the skillet and place it on a metal rack to chill completely.

Nutritional Analysis: Quantity of Energy in Calories: 204, Quantity of Fat: 15g, Quantity of Carbs: 11g, Quantity of Fiber: 3g, Quantity of Protein: 7g

131. Zucchini Walnut Bread

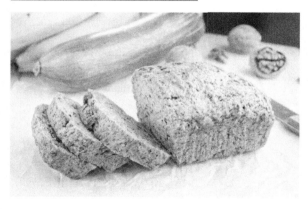

Making and Duration Time: 16 minutes
Cooking Duration: 55 minutes **Number of Portions:** 12

Required Material for this Recipe:
- Almond flour, two tablespoons
- One-fourth cup of coconut flour
- Baking soda, one teaspoon
- Baking powder, 1/2 teaspoon
- A dash of cinnamon powder
- 3 eggs, 1/4 teaspoons of salt
- 1/4 cup unsweetened apple juice

- 1/2 tsp. honey
- Coconut oil, softened, about a quarter cup
- Half a courgetti, sliced
- Walnuts, chopped, about a half a cup

Step By Step Instructions for Recipe:
1. Prepare a 350°F oven. Grease a 9-by-5-inch bread pan.
2. Combine coconut flour, almond flour, baking powder, salt, baking soda, and cinnamon.
3. In a separate dish, combine the beaten eggs, applesauce, honey, and heated coconut oil.
4. Add the liquid components to the dry ones, then mix everything together.
5. Mix in courgetti shreds and walnut pieces.
6. To the ready bread plate, add the mixture.
7. Keep cooking until a probe put in the center comes out clean, 4-50 minutes.
8. After ten minutes, remove the bread from the skillet and place it on a metal rack to chill completely.

Nutritional Analysis: Quantity of Energy in Calories: 212, Quantity of Fat: 16g, Quantity of Carbs: 11g, Quantity of Fiber: 3g, Quantity of Protein: 7g

132. Rosemary Garlic Almond Flour Bread

Making and Duration Time: 11 minutes
Cooking Duration: 30 minutes **Number of Portions:** 10

Required Material for this Recipe:
- Almond flour, two tablespoons
- Coconut flour, two tablespoons; baking powder, two teaspoons
- Salt, 1 teaspoon
- 3 eggs
- Almond milk, sugar-free, 1/4 cup
- Olive oil, 2 tablespoons
- A clove of garlic, minced
- 1 tablespoon of freshly chopped rosemary

Step By Step Instructions for Recipe:
1. Prepare a 350°F oven. Grease a 9-by-5-inch bread pan.
2. In a dish, combine the almond flour, coconut flour, baking soda, and salt.
3. In a separate dish, combine the eggs, almond milk, and olive oil.

4. Add the liquid components to the dry ones, then mix everything together.
5. Mix in some sliced rosemary and garlic.
6. To the ready bread plate, add the mixture.
7. A skewer placed in the middle should come out clear after 25 to 30 minutes of cooking time.
8. After ten minutes, remove the bread from the skillet and place it on a metal rack to chill completely.

Nutritional Analysis: Quantity of Energy in Calories: 180, Quantity of Fat: 15g, Quantity of Carbs: 6g, Quantity of Fiber: 3g, Quantity of Protein: 7g

133. Blueberry Lemon Almond Flour Bread

Making and Duration Time: 14 minutes **Cooking Duration:** 50 minutes **Number of Portions:** 12

Required Material for this Recipe:
- Almond flour, two tablespoons
- One-fourth cup of coconut flour
- Baking flour, one teaspoon
- Baking powder, 1/2 teaspoon
- 3 eggs, 1/4 teaspoon of salt
- 1/4 cup unsweetened apple juice
- 1/2 tsp. honey
- Coconut oil, softened, about a quarter cup
- A pinch of ground ginger
- Blueberries, raw, 1/2 cup

Step By Step Instructions for Recipe:
1. Prepare a 350°F oven. Grease a 9-by-5-inch bread pan.
2. In a dish, combine the almond flour, coconut flour, baking powder, baking soda, and salt.
3. In a separate dish, combine the beaten eggs, applesauce, honey, and heated coconut oil.
4. Add the liquid components to the dry ones, then mix everything together.
5. Fresh blackberries and lemon flavor.
6. To the ready bread plate, add the mixture.
7. Keep cooking until a skewer put in the center comes out clean, 4-5 minutes.
8. After ten minutes, remove the bread from the skillet.

9. Place it on a metal rack to chill completely.

Nutritional Analysis: Quantity of Energy in Calories: 188, Quantity of Fat: 14g, Quantity of Carbs: 11g, Quantity of Fiber: 3g, Quantity of Protein: 6g

134. Zucchini & Banana Loaf

Making and Duration Time: 15 minutes **Cooking Duration:** 50 minutes **Number of Portions:** 12

Required Material for this Recipe:
- Almond flour, two tablespoons
- 1teaspoon of (half) baking soda, (half) baking powder
- A pinch of salt
- Two mature bananas, pureed.
- 1 cup of shredded, drained zucchini
- Two eggs and a quarter cup of heated coconut oil
- One vanilla essence teaspoon
- a pinch of spice, cinnamon
- A pinch of nutmeg, about a quarter teaspoon

Step By Step Instructions for Recipe:
1. Prepare a 350°F oven. Grease a 9-by-5-inch bread pan.
2. Almond flour, baking powder, baking soda, and salt should be combined in a dish.
3. In a separate dish, combine pureed bananas, shredded zucchini, warmed coconut oil, eggs, vanilla essence, cinnamon, and nutmeg.
4. Add the liquid components to the dry ones, then mix everything together.
5. To the ready bread plate, add the mixture.
6. Keep cooking until a skewer put in the center comes out clean, about 4-50 minutes.
7. After ten minutes, remove the bread from the skillet.
8. Place it on a metal rack to chill completely.

Nutritional Analysis: Quantity of Energy in Calories: 186, Quantity of Fat: 14g, Quantity of Carbs: 10g, Quantity of Fiber: 3g, Quantity of Protein: 6g.

135. Chocolate Chip Coconut Flour Bread

Making and Duration Time: 14 minutes **Cooking Duration:** 45 minutes **Number of Portions:** 12

Required Material for this Recipe:
- One-half cup of coconut flour
- A pinch of baking soda
- 1/4 teaspoon of salt
- 6 eggs
- Coconut oil, softened, about a quarter cup
- One-fourth cup of maple syrup
- Almond milk, sugar-free, 1/4 cup
- One vanilla essence teaspoon
- A half cup of semisweet chocolate chunks

Step By Step Instructions for Recipe:
1. Prepare a 350°F oven. Grease a 9-by-5-inch bread pan.
2. In a dish, combine the coconut flour, baking soda, and salt.
3. In a separate dish, combine eggs with warmed coconut oil, maple syrup, almond milk, and vanilla.
4. Add the liquid components to the dry ones, then mix everything together.
5. Mix in some mini dark chocolate chunks.
6. To the ready bread plate, add the mixture.
7. A skewer placed in the middle should come out clear after about 40 to 45 minutes of cooking time.
8. After ten minutes, remove the bread from the skillet and place it on a metal rack to chill completely.

Nutritional Analysis: Quantity of Energy in Calories: 178, Quantity of Fat: 12g, Quantity of Carbs: 13g, Quantity of Fiber: 4g, Quantity of Protein: 6g

136. Carrot Raisin Loaf

Making and Duration Time: 15 minutes **Cooking Duration:** 45 minutes **Number of Portions:** 12

Required Material for this Recipe:
- Almond flour, two tablespoons
- 1 teaspoon (half of each) of baking soda and baking powder
- A pinch of salt
- Carrots, grated: 2 quarts
- 1/2 cups of dried fruit (raisins)
- a quarter cup of heated coconut oil, 3 eggs
- One vanilla essence teaspoon
- one-fourth of a teaspoon of spice (cinnamon and nutmeg)

Step By Step Instructions for Recipe:
1. Prepare a 350°F oven. Grease a 9-by-5-inch bread pan.
2. In a dish, combine the almond flour, baking powder, baking soda, and salt.
3. In a different dish, combine shredded carrots, raisins, warmed coconut oil, eggs, vanilla essence, cinnamon, and nutmeg.
4. Add the liquid components to the dry ones, then mix everything together.
5. To the ready bread plate, add the mixture.
6. Bake until a knife stuck in the middle comes out clean, about 40 to 45 minutes.
7. After ten minutes, remove the bread from the skillet and place it on a metal rack to chill completely.

Nutritional Analysis: Quantity of Energy in Calories: 201, Quantity of Fat: 15g, Quantity of Carbs: 11g, Quantity of Fiber: 4g, Quantity of Protein: 6g

137. Blueberry & Lemon Loaf

Making and Duration Time: 15 minutes **Cooking Duration:** 45 minutes **Number of Portions:** 12

Required Material for this Recipe:
- Almond flour, two tablespoons
- 1 teaspoon (half of each) of baking soda and baking powder
- A pinch of salt
- Blueberries, raw, 1/2 cup
- a quarter cup of heated coconut oil, three eggs
- A pinch of lemon juice and rind and a pinch of salt
- One vanilla essence teaspoon

Step By Step Instructions for Recipe:
1. Prepare a 350°F oven. Grease a 9-by-5-inch bread pan.
2. In a dish, combine the almond flour, baking powder, baking soda, and salt.

3. In a separate dish, combine blueberries, coconut oil, eggs, lemon peel, lemon juice, and vanilla essence.
4. Add the liquid components to the dry ones, then mix everything together.
5. To the ready bread plate, add the mixture.
6. Bake until a knife stuck in the middle comes out clear, about 40 to 45 minutes.
7. After ten minutes, remove the bread from the skillet and place it on a metal rack to chill completely.

Nutritional Analysis: Quantity of Energy in Calories: 186, Quantity of Fat: 15g, Quantity of Carbs: 8g, Quantity of Fiber: 3g, Quantity of Protein: 6g

138. Pumpkin Spice Loaf

Making and Duration Time: 15 minutes
Cooking Duration: 45 minutes **Number of Portions:** 12

Required Material for this Recipe:
- Almond flour, two tablespoons
- Baking powder, 1/2 teaspoon
- A pinch of baking soda
- 1/4 teaspoon pepper
- Pureed pumpkin, one cup
- a quarter cup of heated coconut oil, three eggs
- a pinch of spice
- Add 1/2 tsp cinnamon
- Ground Ginger, 14 Teaspoon
- a pinch of powdered garlic

Step By Step Instructions for Recipe:
1. Prepare a 350°F oven. Grease a 9-by-5-inch bread pan.
2. In a dish, combine the almond flour, baking powder, baking soda, and salt.
3. In a separate dish, combine the warmed coconut oil, pumpkin purée, eggs, vanilla essence, spices (cinnamon, nutmeg, ginger, and cloves), and salt.
4. Add the liquid components to the dry ones, then mix everything together.
5. To the ready bread plate, add the mixture.
6. Bake until a knife stuck in the middle comes out clean, about 40 to 45 minutes.

7. After ten minutes, remove the bread from the skillet and place it on a metal rack to chill completely.

Nutritional Analysis: Quantity of Energy in Calories: 190, Quantity of Fat: 15g, Quantity of Carbs: 9g, Quantity of Fiber: 4g, Quantity of Protein: 6g

139. Chocolate & Zucchini Loaf

Making and Duration Time: 20 minutes
Cooking Duration: 50 minutes **Number of Portions:** 12

Required Material for this Recipe:
- Almond flour, two tablespoons
- 1/4 cup unsweetened chocolate
- Just a tsp of baking soda
- A pinch (1/2 tsp) of baking powder
- 1/4 teaspoon pepper
- The equivalent of 2 tablespoons of shredded zucchini
- Coconut oil, warmed, 1/4 cup
- 3 eggs
- One vanilla essence teaspoon
- 1-fourth of a cup of honey

Step By Step Instructions for Recipe:
1. Prepare a 350°F oven. Grease a 9-by-5-inch bread pan.
2. Add the chocolate powder, baking soda, baking powder, and salt to the almond flour and stir until combined.
3. In a separate dish, combine shredded zucchini with warmed coconut oil, eggs, vanilla, and honey.
4. Add the liquid components to the dry ones, then mix everything together.
5. To the ready bread plate, add the mixture.
6. A skewer placed in the middle should come out clear after 50 minutes of cooking time.
7. After ten minutes, remove the bread from the skillet and place it on a metal rack to chill completely.

Nutritional Analysis: Quantity of Energy in Calories: 206, Quantity of Fat: 15g, Quantity of Carbs: 14g, Quantity of Fiber: 4g, Quantity of Protein: 6g

140. Almond Flour Bread

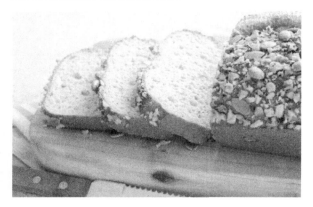

Making and Duration Time: 12 minutes
Cooking Duration: 50 minutes **Number of Portions:** 12

Required Material for this Recipe:
- Almond flour, two cups
- One-fourth cup of coconut flour
- Flaxseeds, 1/4 cup
- Just a 1/2 tsp of baking soda
- a pinch of salt, 5 big eggs
- Coconut oil, softened, about a quarter cup
- Apple cider vinegar, about a tablespoon

Step By Step Instructions for Recipe:
1. Prepare a 350°F oven.
2. To make the batter, combine the coconut flour, almond flour, powdered flaxseed, baking soda, and salt in a large dish.
3. In a separate dish, thoroughly mix the yolks with the coconut oil and the apple cider vinegar.
4. Mix the moist and dry components together in a large bowl.
5. To a ready-made bread plate, pour the mixture.
6. Keep baking until a probe put into the middle of the bread comes out clean, about 45 to 50 minutes.
7. Ten minutes of cooking time is recommended before serving.

Nutritional Analysis: Quantity of Energy in Calories: 188 kcal, Quantity of Fat: 16 g, Quantity of Protein: 7 g, Quantity of Carbs: 6 g, Quantity of Fiber: 4 g

141. Oat Flour Banana Loaf

Making and Duration Time: 10 minutes
Cooking Duration: 45 minutes **Number of Portions:** 12

Required Material for this Recipe:
- Three mature bananas, pureed.
- 2 eggs
- 1/2 tsp. of honey
- Coconut oil, softened, about a quarter cup
- Oat flour, 2 mugs
- Baking flour, one teaspoon
- Baking powder, 1/2 teaspoon
- One-half teaspoon of cinnamon powder
- A little salt

Step By Step Instructions for Recipe:
1. Prepare a 350°F oven.
2. Add the eggs, honey, coconut oil, and vanilla essence to the pureed bananas and stir until combined.
3. In a separate dish, whisk together the wheat flour, baking soda, baking powder, powdered cinnamon, and salt.
4. Mix the moist and dry components together in a large bowl.
5. To a ready-made bread plate, pour the mixture.
6. A skewer placed in the middle should come out clear after 40 to 45 minutes of cooking time.
7. Ten minutes of cooking time is recommended before serving.

Nutritional Analysis: Quantity of Energy in Calories: 164 kcal, Quantity of Fat: 6 g, Quantity of Protein: 5g, Quantity of Carbs: 25 g, Quantity of Fiber: 2 g

142. Flaxseed Bread

Making and Duration Time: 12 minutes
Cooking Duration: 45 minutes **Number of Portions:** 12 slices

Required Material for this Recipe:
- Almond flour, 1 1/2 mugs
- 1/2 of a cup of flaxseed
- One-fourth cup of coconut flour
- One-fourth cup of psyllium pod
- Just a tsp of baking soda

- A pinch of salt
- 4 eggs
- One-fourth cup of olive oil
- Approximately one-half cup of water

Step By Step Instructions for Recipe:
1. Prepare a baking tray with parchment paper and preheat the oven to 350 degrees Fahrenheit.
2. Add the baking soda, salt, and flaxseed to the dish with the almond flour, coconut flour, psyllium fiber, and flaxseed.
3. Eggs, olive oil, and water should be mixed together in a separate dish.
4. Mix the dry and liquid components together until a mixture form.
5. Spread the dough evenly across the bottom of the prepped bread container.
6. A skewer placed in the middle should come out clear after 40 to 45 minutes of cooking time.
7. After ten minutes, remove the bread from the skillet and place it on a metal rack to chill completely.

Nutritional Analysis: Quantity of Energy in Calories: 157, Quantity of Fat: 12g, Quantity of Carbs: 7g, Quantity of Fiber: 5g, Quantity of Protein: 6g

143. Gluten-Free Zucchini Bread

Making and Duration Time: 17 minutes **Cooking Duration:** 1-hour **Number of Portions:** 10

Required Material for this Recipe:
- Almond flour, two mugs
- One-half cup of coconut flour
- Just a half tsp of baking powder, 1 tsp of baking soda
- A pinch of salt
- 2. tsp of cinnamon
- Add 1/2 tsp cinnamon
- Melted coconut oil equals 1/2 cup
- Raw Honey, 1/2 Cup
- 3 eggs
- One vanilla essence teaspoon
- Half a courgette, sliced

Step By Step Instructions for Recipe:
1. Prepare a 350°F oven. Spread coconut oil on a bread griddle.

2. Almond flour, coconut flour, baking soda, baking powder, salt, cinnamon, and nutmeg should all be combined in one dish.
3. In a separate dish, combine the coconut oil with the honey, eggs, and vanilla.
4. Mix the liquid and dry components together in a large bowl. Stir in the zucchini gratings.
5. To the ready bread plate, add the mixture.
6. A skewer placed in the center should come out clear after 1 hour of cooking time.
7. Ten minutes of chilling time and then transfer to a wire rack.

Nutritional Analysis: Quantity of Energy in Calories: 320, Quantity of Fat: 23g, Quantity of Protein: 8g, Quantity of Carbs: 23g, Quantity of Fiber: 6g

144. Buckwheat and Chia Seed Loaf

Making and Duration Time: 11 minutes **Cooking Duration:** 40 minutes **Number of Portions:** 12

Required Material for this Recipe:
- One and a half cups of buckwheat flour
- Just half cup of tapioca flour
- Chia seeds, about half a cup
- Baking powder, 2 teaspoons
- 1 teaspoon of salt
- One-fourth cup of olive oil
- A glass (250ml) of Water
- 3 eggs

Step By Step Instructions for Recipe:
1. Prepare a 350°F oven. Spread olive oil in a bread tin.
2. Put the chia seeds, baking powder, and salt in a dish with buckwheat flour and tapioca flour.
3. Eggs, water, and olive oil should be combined in a separate dish.
4. Combine the moist and dry components in a large mixing bowl.
5. To the ready bread plate, add the mixture.
6. Wait 40 minutes or until a skewer put in the center comes out clear.
7. Ten minutes of chilling time and then transfer to a wire rack.

Nutritional Analysis: Quantity of Energy in Calories: 144, Quantity of Fat: 8g, Quantity of Protein: 4g, Quantity of Carbs: 16g, Quantity of Fiber: 4g

145. Gluten-free Seed Bread

Making and Duration Time: 17 minutes
Cooking Duration: 1-hour **Number of Portions:** 10 slices

Required Material for this Recipe:
- Almond flour measuring a cup, same proportion of sunflower seeds
- Roasted Pumpkin Seeds, Half a Cup
- Flaxseeds, to the amount of a half cup
- A quarter cup of chia seeds
- An equal amount of sesame seeds, about a quarter cup
- Psyllium peel, 2 tablespoons
- 1 teaspoon of salt
- 3 eggs
- One-fourth cup of olive oil
- A glass of water (250ml)

Step By Step Instructions for Recipe:
1. Preheat the oven to 350 degrees Fahrenheit and line a baking tray with parchment paper.
2. In a large dish, mix together all the dry ingredients.
3. Eggs, olive oil, and water should be mixed together in a separate dish.
4. Combine the moist and dry components in a large mixing bowl.
5. Spread the ingredients out on the baking tray that has been greased.
6. A skewer placed in the center should come out clear after 1 hour of cooking time.
7. Ten minutes of chilling time and then transfer to a wire rack.
8. Serve.

Nutritional Information per slice: Quantity of Energy in Calories: 242, Quantity of Fat: 20g, Quantity of Carbs: 10g, Quantity of Fiber: 7g, Quantity of Protein: 9g

146. Buckwheat Banana Loaf

Making and Duration Time: 16 minutes
Cooking Duration: 50 minutes **Number of Portions:** 10 slices

Required Material for this Recipe:
- Fruits: 2 big bananas
- 1-quarter cup of honey
- one-fourth cup of coconut oil
- Exactly two eggs
- Cup of buckwheat flour, 1 teaspoon of baking powder, 1 teaspoon of vanilla essence
- a pinch of spice, cinnamon
- 1/4 teaspoon pepper

Step By Step Instructions for Recipe:
1. Prepare a baking tray with coconut oil and preheat the oven to 350°F.
2. The bananas should be mashed until they are completely smooth.
3. Put the honey, coconut oil, eggs, and vanilla essence in a dish and mix them together thoroughly with a spatula.
4. In a separate dish, mix the baking soda, cinnamon, buckwheat flour, and pepper.
5. Put the liquids into the dry and stir until everything is incorporated. Put the mixture on the pan and level it off with a spoon.
6. A skewer placed in the center should come out clear after 45–50 minutes of cooking time. Ten minutes later, transfer to a wire receptacle to chill completely.

Nutritional Information per slice: Quantity of Energy in Calories: 160, Quantity of Fat: 6g, Quantity of Carbs: 24g, Quantity of Fiber: 3g, Quantity of Protein: 3g

147. Coconut Flour Loaf

Making and Duration Time: 12 minutes
Cooking Duration: 50 minutes **Number of Portions:** 12 slices

Required Material for this Recipe:
- One-half cup of coconut flour
- Half cup of flaxseed meal
- Psyllium peel, 1/2 cup
- Baking powder, one teaspoon
- 8 big eggs and 1/2 tsp of salt

- Coconut oil, softened, about a quarter cup
- Approximately one-half cup of water

Step By Step Instructions for Recipe:

1. Prepare a 350°F oven. Combine the psyllium husk powder, salt, powdered flaxseed, coconut flour, and baking powder in a dish.
2. Combine the water, coconut oil, and yolks in a dish and stir until smooth.
3. Spread the mixture out evenly on the prepped baking tray.
4. Bake the bread for 50–55 minutes, or until a skewer put in the center comes out clear.
5. Ten minutes later, transfer to a wire receptacle to chill completely. Serve.

Nutritional Information (1 slice): Quantity of Energy in Calories: 125, Quantity of Fat: 9g, Carbohydrate: 6g, Quantity of Fiber: 4g, Quantity of Protein: 6g

148. Buckwheat Flour Loaf

Making and Duration Time: 15 minutes **Cooking Duration:** one-hour **Number of Portions:** 12 slices

Required Material for this Recipe:

- Buckwheat flour, three tablespoons
- One-half cup of coconut flour
- Half of a cup of flaxseed meal
- Just a pinch of baking powder
- 1/4 teaspoon pepper
- 6 eggs
- A half cup of olive oil
- Almond milk, sugar-free, 1/2 cup
- Two tablespoons of honey

Step By Step Instructions for Recipe:

1. Prepare a 350°F oven.
2. In a dish, whisk together the buckwheat flour, coconut flour, powdered flaxseed, baking soda, and salt.
3. In a separate dish, whisk together the eggs, olive oil, almond milk, and honey.
4. Put the liquids into the dry and stir until everything is incorporated.
5. Spread the ingredients evenly in a baking pan that has been oiled.
6. A skewer placed in the center should come out clear after 1 hour of cooking time.
7. Ten minutes later, transfer to a wire receptacle to chill completely. Serve

Nutritional Analysis: Quantity of Energy in Calories: 201, Quantity of Fat: 12g, Quantity of Carbs: 20g, Quantity of Fiber: 8g, Quantity of Protein: 6g

CHAPTER 9: SMOOTHIE RECIPES

149. Pineapple Turmeric Smoothie

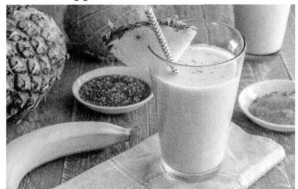

Making and Duration Time: 7 minutes **Number of Portions:** 1

Required Material for this Recipe:
- Pineapple pieces, enough for a cup
- Coconut milk, half a cup
- Turmeric, powdered, 1/2 teaspoon
- Ginger, minced, 1/2 teaspoon
- Cinnamon, powdered, 1/4 teaspoon
- Half a banana
- A Pinch of Pepper
- Ice, 1/2 cup

Step By Step Instructions for Recipe:
1. Put everything in a blender and blend until it's smooth.
2. Serve the drink in tumblers by pouring them in.

Nutritional Analysis: Quantity of Energy in Calories: 246, Quantity of Fat: 19g, Quantity of Carbs: 20g, Quantity of Fiber: 3g, Quantity of Protein: 3g

150. Mixed Berry Chia Seed Smoothie

Making and Duration Time: 7 minutes **Number of Portions:** 1

Required Material for this Recipe:
- One cup of chilled berry blend
- Water from half coconut

- Half a banana
- A tablespoon of chia seeds
- Vanilla essence, 1/2 teaspoon
- Ice, 1/2 cup

Step By Step Instructions for Recipe:
1. Put everything in a blender and blend until it's smooth.
2. Serve it in a glass by pouring it out.

Nutritional Analysis: Quantity of Energy in Calories: 182, Quantity of Fat: 3g, Quantity of Carbs: 38g, Quantity of Fiber: 11g, Quantity of Protein: 4g

151. Mango Ginger Smoothie

Making and Duration Time: 7 minutes **Number of Portions:** 1

Required Material for this Recipe:
- Frozen mango cubes, about a cup
- Coconut milk, half a cup
- Half a banana
- Ginger, minced, 1/2 teaspoon
- Turmeric powder, 1/2 teaspoon
- Ice, 1/2 cup

Step By Step Instructions for Recipe:
1. Put everything in a blender and blend until it's smooth.
2. Serve it in a glass by pouring it out.

Nutritional Analysis: Quantity of Energy in Calories: 208, Quantity of Fat: 12g, Quantity of Carbs: 24g, Quantity of Fiber: 3g, Quantity of Protein: 2g

152. Blueberry Avocado Smoothie

Making and Duration Time: 5 minutes **Number of Portions:** 1

Required Material for this Recipe:
- Frozen blackberries, one cup
- Avocado, just half

- Almond milk, sugar-free, 1/2 cup
- Ginger, minced, 1/2 teaspoon
- One-half teaspoon of cinnamon powder
- Ice, 1/2 cup

Step By Step Instructions for Recipe:
1. Put everything in a blender and blend until it's smooth.
2. Serve it in a glass by pouring it out.

Nutritional Analysis: Quantity of Energy in Calories: 259, Quantity of Fat: 19g, Quantity of Carbs: 22g, Quantity of Fiber: 9g, Quantity of Protein: 4g

153. Green Tea Berry Smoothie
Making and Duration Time: 7 minutes **Number of Portions:** 1

Required Material for this Recipe:
- One cup of chilled berry blend
- Green tea, made and cooled, half a cup
- Half a pineapple
- Ginger, minced, 1/2 teaspoon
- 12 teaspoons of honey
- Ice, 1/2 cup

Step By Step Instructions for Recipe:
1. Put everything in a blender and blend until it's smooth.
2. Serve it in a glass by pouring it out.

Nutritional Analysis: Quantity of Energy in Calories: 158, Quantity of Fat: 0g, Quantity of Carbs: 40g, Quantity of Fiber: 6g, Quantity of Protein: 2g

154. Cucumber Ginger Smoothie

Making and Duration Time: 6 minutes **Number of Portions:** 1

Required Material for this Recipe:
- 1/2 of a big cucumber, sliced
- Almond milk, sugar-free, 1/2 cup
- Half a banana
- Ginger, minced, 1/2 teaspoon
- 1/2 teaspoon of honey
- Ice, 1/2 cup

Step By Step Instructions for Recipe:
1. Put everything in a blender and blend until it's smooth.
2. Serve it in a glass by pouring it out.

Nutritional Analysis: Quantity of Energy in Calories: 108, Quantity of Fat: 1g, Quantity of Carbs: 27g, Quantity of Fiber: 3g, Quantity of Protein: 2g

155. Pineapple Turmeric Smoothie

Making and Duration Time: 6 minutes **Number of Portions:** 1

Required Material for this Recipe:
- Frozen pineapple pieces, about a mug
- Coconut milk, half a cup
- Half a banana
- Turmeric powder, 1/2 teaspoon
- Ginger, minced, 1/2 teaspoon
- Ice, 1/2 cup

Step By Step Instructions for Recipe:
1. Put everything in a blender and blend until it's smooth.
2. Serve it in a glass by pouring it out.

Nutritional Analysis: Quantity of Energy in Calories: 208, Quantity of Fat: 12g, Quantity of Carbs: 24g, Quantity of Fiber: 3g, Quantity of Protein: 2g

156. Cherry Almond Smoothie

Making and Duration Time: 7 minutes **Number of Portions:** 1

Required Material for this Recipe:
- Frozen cherries in a cup
- Almond milk, sugar-free, 1/2 cup
- Half a banana
- 1/2 teaspoon of honey
- a pinch of almond essence, 1/4 tsp
- Ice, 1/2 cup

Step By Step Instructions for Recipe:
1. Put everything in a blender and blend until it's smooth.
2. Serve it in a glass by pouring it out.

Nutritional Analysis: Quantity of Energy in Calories: 173, Quantity of Fat: 3g, Quantity of Carbs: 37g, Quantity of Fiber: 5g, Quantity of Protein: 3g

157. Blueberry Beet Smoothie

Making and Duration Time: 5 minutes **Number of Portions:** 1

Required Material for this Recipe:
- The equivalent of a half cup of frozen Blueberry
- 1/2 cups of diced, boiled beet
- Almond milk, sugar-free, 1/2 cup
- Half a banana
- 1/2 teaspoon of honey
- Ice, 1/2 cup

Step By Step Instructions for Recipe:
1. Put everything in a blender and blend until it's smooth.
2. Serve it in a glass by pouring it out.

Nutritional Analysis: Quantity of Energy in Calories: 178, Quantity of Fat: 2g, Quantity of Carbs: 40g, Quantity of Fiber: 7g, Quantity of Protein: 3g

158. Mango Ginger Smoothie

Making and Duration Time: 7 minutes **Number of Portions:** 1

Required Material for this Recipe:
- Frozen mango cubes, about a mug
- Coconut milk, half a cup
- Half a banana
- Ginger, minced, 1/2 teaspoon
- 1/2 teaspoon of honey
- Ice, 1/2 cup

Step By Step Instructions for Recipe:
1. Put everything in a blender and blend until it's smooth.
2. Serve it in a glass by pouring it out.

Nutritional Analysis: Quantity of Energy in Calories: 232, Quantity of Fat: 14g, Quantity of Carbs: 28g, Quantity of Fiber: 3g, Quantity of Protein: 2g

159. Raspberry Chocolate Smoothie

Making and Duration Time: 5 minutes **Number of Portions:** 1

Required Material for this Recipe:
- Frozen raspberries in a cup
- Almond milk, sugar-free, 1/2 cup
- Half a banana
- Cocoa powder, 1 tablespoon
- 1/2 teaspoon of honey
- Ice, 1/2 cup

Step By Step Instructions for Recipe:
Put everything in a blender and blend until it's smooth.
Serve it in a glass by pouring it out.

Nutritional Analysis: Quantity of Energy in Calories: 156, Quantity of Fat: 2g, Quantity of Carbs: 34g, Quantity of Fiber: 11g, Quantity of Protein: 4g

160. Spinach Avocado Smoothie

Making and Duration Time: 7 minutes **Number of Portions:** 1

Required Material for this Recipe:
- One cup of Spinach
- Just half avocado
- Almond milk, sugar-free, 1/2 cup
- Half a banana
- 1/2 teaspoon of honey
- Ice, half a cup

Step By Step Instructions for Recipe:
1. Put everything in a blender and blend until it's smooth.
2. Serve it in a glass by pouring it out.

Nutritional Analysis: Quantity of Energy in Calories: 242, Quantity of Fat: 16g, Quantity of Carbs: 25g, Quantity of Fiber: 8g, Quantity of Protein: 4g

161. Carrot Ginger Smoothie

Making and Duration Time: 5 minutes **Number of Portions:** 1

Required Material for this Recipe:
- Carrot Juice, 0.5 Cups
- Almond milk, sugar-free, 1/2 cup

- Half a banana
- Ginger, minced, 1/2 teaspoon
- 1/2 teaspoon of honey
- Ice, 1/2 cup

Step By Step Instructions for Recipe:
1. Put everything in a blender and blend until it's smooth.
2. Serve it in a glass by pouring it out.

Nutritional Analysis: Quantity of Energy in Calories: 137, Quantity of Fat: 2g, Quantity of Carbs: 32g, Quantity of Fiber: 2g, Quantity of Protein: 2g

162. Peach Almond Smoothie

Making and Duration Time: 7 minutes **Number of Portions:** 1

Required Material for this Recipe:
- Frozen peach, a cup
- Almond milk, sugar-free, 1/2 cup
- Half a banana
- 1/2 teaspoon of honey
- a pinch of almond essence, 1/4 tsp
- Ice, 1/2 cup

Step By Step Instructions for Recipe:
1. Put everything in a blender and blend until it's smooth.
2. Serve it in a glass by pouring it out.

Nutritional Analysis: Quantity of Energy in Calories: 172, Quantity of Fat: 3g, Quantity of Carbs: 36g, Quantity of Fiber: 4g, Quantity of Protein: 3g

163. Blueberry Flaxseed Smoothie

Making and Duration Time: 5 minutes **Number of Portions:** 1

Required Material for this Recipe:
- Frozen blueberries, one mug
- Almond milk, sugar-free, 1/2 cup
- Just half banana
- Ground flaxseed, 1 tablespoon
- 1/2 teaspoon of honey
- Ice, 1/2 cup

Step By Step Instructions for Recipe:
1. Put everything in a blender and blend until it's smooth.

2. Serve it in a glass by pouring it out.

Nutritional Analysis: Quantity of Energy in Calories: 214, Quantity of Fat: 6g, Quantity of Carbs: 39g, Quantity of Fiber: 8g, Quantity of Protein: 4g

164. Tropical Turmeric Smoothie

Making and Duration Time: 5 minutes **Number of Portions:** 1

Required Material for this Recipe:
- Pineapple chunks, frozen, 1 cup
- Coconut milk, sugar-free, 1/2 cup
- Half a banana
- Turmeric powder, 1/2 teaspoon
- 1/2 teaspoon of honey
- Ice, 1/2 cup

Step By Step Instructions for Recipe:
1. Put everything in a blender and blend until it's smooth.
2. Serve it in a glass by pouring it out.

Nutritional Analysis: Quantity of Energy in Calories: 181, Quantity of Fat: 4g, Quantity of Carbs: 38g, Quantity of Fiber: 4g, Quantity of Protein: 2g

165. Mango Chia Smoothie

Making and Duration Time: 5 minutes **Number of Portions:** 1

Required Material for this Recipe:
- One cold fruit serving
- Almond milk, sugar-free, 1/2 cup
- Half a pineapple
- Chia nuts, 1 tablespoon
- 12 teaspoons of honey
- Ice, 1/2 cup

Step By Step Instructions for Recipe:
1. Put everything in a blender and blend until it's smooth.
2. Serve it in a glass by pouring it out.

Nutritional Analysis: Quantity of Energy in Calories: 210, Quantity of Fat: 6g, Quantity of Carbs: 38g, Quantity of Fiber: 7g, Quantity of Protein: 3

166. Kale Pineapple Smoothie

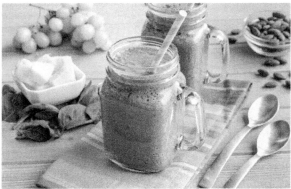

Making and Duration Time: 5 minutes **Number of Portions:** 1

Required Material for this Recipe:
- One cup of finely minced greens (kale)
- Pineapple, refrigerated, 1/2 cup
- Just half banana
- Almond milk, sugar-free, 1/2 cup
- 1/2 teaspoon of honey
- Ice, 1/2 cup

Step By Step Instructions for Recipe:
1. Put everything in a blender and blend until it's smooth.
2. Serve it in a glass by pouring it out.

Nutritional Analysis: Quantity of Energy in Calories: 161, Quantity of Fat: 3g, Quantity of Carbs: 33g, Quantity of Fiber: 4g, Quantity of Protein: 5g

167. Raspberry Almond Butter Smoothie

Making and Duration Time: 5 minutes **Number of Portions:** 1

Required Material for this Recipe:
- Frozen raspberries in a cup
- Half a banana
- Almond butter, one tablespoon
- Almond milk, sugar-free, 1/2 cup
- 12 teaspoons of honey
- Ice, 1/2 cup

Step By Step Instructions for Recipe:
1. Put everything in a blender and blend until it's smooth.
2. Serve it in a glass by pouring it out.

Nutritional Analysis: Quantity of Energy in Calories: 234, Quantity of Fat: 10g, Quantity of Carbs: 34g, Quantity of Fiber: 12g, Quantity of Protein: 5g

168. Pear Turmeric Smoothie

Making and Duration Time: 5 minutes **Number of Portions:** 1

Required Material for this Recipe:
- Frozen pears in a cup
- Half a banana
- Turmeric powder, 1/2 teaspoon
- Almond milk, sugar-free, 1/2 cup
- 1/2 teaspoon of honey
- Ice, 1/2 cup

Step By Step Instructions for Recipe:
1. Put everything in a blender and blend until it's smooth.
2. Serve it in a glass by pouring it out.

Nutritional Analysis: Quantity of Energy in Calories: 176, Quantity of Fat: 3g, Quantity of Carbs: 36g, Quantity of Fiber: 4g, Quantity of Protein: 3g

169. Cucumber Mint Smoothie

Making and Duration Time: 5 minutes **Number of Portions:** 1

Required Material for this Recipe:
- Cucumber, diced, one cup
- Pineapple, refrigerated, 1/2 cup, and 1/2 banana
- One-fourth cup of mint stems
- Almond milk, sugar-free, 1/2 cup
- 1/2 teaspoon of honey
- Ice, 1/2 cup

Step By Step Instructions for Recipe:
1. Put everything in a blender and blend until it's smooth.
2. Serve it in a glass by pouring it out.

Nutritional Analysis: Quantity of Energy in Calories: 157, Quantity of Fat: 3g, Quantity of Carbs: 32g, Quantity of Fiber: 5g, Quantity of Protein: 4g

170. Mango Ginger Smoothie

Making and Duration Time: 5 minutes **Number of Portions:** 1

Required Material for this Recipe:
- One cold fruit serving
- Half a banana
- Ginger, minced, 1/2 teaspoon
- Almond milk, sugar-free, 1/2 cup
- 12 teaspoons of honey
- Ice, 1/2 cup

Step By Step Instructions for Recipe:
1. Put everything in a blender and blend until it's smooth.
2. Serve it in a glass by pouring it out.

Nutritional Analysis: Quantity of Energy in Calories: 178, Quantity of Fat: 3g, Quantity of Carbs: 37g, Quantity of Fiber: 4g, Quantity of Protein: 3g

171. Blackberry Spinach Smoothie

Making and Duration Time: 5 minutes **Number of Portions:** 1

Required Material for this Recipe:
- Frozen blackberries, one cup
- Just one cup of baby Spinach
- Half a banana
- Almond milk, sugar-free, 1/2 cup
- 1/2 teaspoon of honey
- Ice, 1/2 cup

Step By Step Instructions for Recipe:
1. Put everything in a blender and blend until it's smooth.
2. Serve it in a glass by pouring it out.

Nutritional Analysis: Quantity of Energy in Calories: 160, Quantity of Fat: 3g, Quantity of Carbs: 34g, Quantity of Fiber: 6g, Quantity of Protein: 4g

172. Peanut Butter Banana Smoothie

Making and Duration Time: 5 minutes **Number of Portions:** 1

Required Material for this Recipe:
- Single Banana
- Two tablespoons of peanut butter
- Almond milk, sugar-free, 1/2 cup
- 12 teaspoons of honey
- Ice, 1/2 cup

Step By Step Instructions for Recipe:
1. Put everything in a blender and blend until it's smooth.
2. Serve it in a glass by pouring it out.

Nutritional Analysis: Quantity of Energy in Calories: 230, Quantity of Fat: 10g, Quantity of Carbs: 33g, Quantity of Fiber: 4g, Quantity of Protein: 7g

173. Pineapple Turmeric Smoothie

Making and Duration Time: 5 minutes **Number of Portions:** 1

Required Material for this Recipe:
- Pineapple chunks, frozen, in a cup
- Turmeric powder, 1/2 teaspoon
- Almond milk, sugar-free, 1/2 cup
- 1/2 teaspoon of honey
- Ice, 1/2 cup

Step By Step Instructions for Recipe:
1. Put everything in a blender and blend until it's smooth.
2. Serve it in a glass by pouring it out.

Nutritional Analysis: Quantity of Energy in Calories: 133, Quantity of Fat: 3g, Quantity of Carbs: 29g, Quantity of Fiber: 2g, Quantity of Protein: 2g

CHAPTER 10: VEGGIE RECIPE

174. Roasted Turmeric Cauliflower

Making and Duration Time: 10 minutes
Cooking Duration: 25 minutes **Number of Portions:** 4

Required Material for this Recipe:
- Flowers from a cauliflower stem
- Olive oil, 2 tablespoons
- Ground turmeric, 1 teaspoon
- Ground cumin, 1 teaspoon
- Pepper and salt

Step By Step Instructions for Recipe:
1. Turn the oven on to 400 degrees.
2. Olive oil, turmeric, cumin, salt, pepper, and cauliflower pieces should be combined in a dish.
3. Toss the vegetables to evenly coat them.
4. Cauliflower should be baked at 400 degrees for 25 minutes until it is browned and soft. Serve

Nutritional Analysis: Quantity of Energy in Calories: 95, Quantity of Fat: 7g, Quantity of Carbs: 8g, Quantity of Fiber: 3g, Quantity of Protein: 3g

175. Spinach and Mushroom Stir-Fry

Making and Duration Time: 13 minutes
Cooking Duration: 15 minutes **Number of Portions:** 4

Required Material for this Recipe:
- 2 teaspoons butter
- Two bulbs of chopped garlic
- Mushrooms, cut (8 ounces)
- 4.25 ounces of baby greens
- Soy sauce and honey, just 1 tbsp of each
- Pepper and salt

Step By Step Instructions for Recipe:
1. Olive oil should be warmed over medium heat in a pan.
2. Cook the garlic for 1-2 minutes or until it starts to smell good.
3. Slice the mushrooms and bake them for 5–7 minutes or until they are tender.

4. Stir in some fresh greens and cook it for a couple of minutes at a low boil.
5. Whisk honey and soy sauce together.
6. Stir-fry the vegetables for 2–3 minutes after adding the marinade.
7. Season with salt and pepper, then serve.

Nutritional Analysis: Quantity of Energy in Calories: 67, Quantity of Fat: 4g, Quantity of Carbs: 8g, Quantity of Fiber: 2g, Quantity of Protein: 3g

176. Turmeric Lentil Soup with Cumin

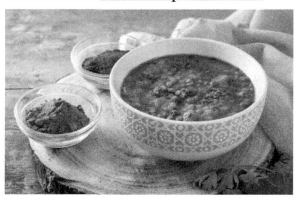

Making and Duration Time: 11 minutes
Cooking Duration: 30 minutes **Number of Portions:** 6

Required Material for this Recipe:
- Approximately one tablespoon of olive oil
- One small shallot, minced
- Two, chopped garlic
- Two carrots, sliced
- Two celery stems, sliced
- Ground turmeric, 1 teaspoon
- Ground cumin, 1 teaspoon
- One teaspoon of cilantro powder
- Red legumes (Lentils), one cup uncooked, soaked, and strained
- Vegetable Stock, 4 Cups
- Pepper and salt

Step By Step Instructions for Recipe:
1. Olive oil should be warmed over medium heat in a saucepan.

2. Put the garlic and shallot in and roast for 2 to 3 minutes or until the shallot is soft and the garlic is aromatic.
3. Toss in some diced carrots and celery, then pop it in the oven for about 5 minutes.
4. Turmeric, cumin, and cilantro seeds should be mixed with the soil.
5. Add dehydrated legumes and veggie stock to the saucepan.
6. To make the lentils tender, bring the broth to a boil, then reduce the heat and let it stew for 20–25 minutes.
7. Season with salt and pepper, then serve.

Nutritional Analysis: Quantity of Energy in Calories: 150, Quantity of Fat: 3g, Quantity of Carbs: 24g, Quantity of Fiber: 10g, Quantity of Protein: 9g

177. Quinoa Salad with Tomatoes and Avocado

Making and Duration Time: 10 minutes **Cooking Duration:** 17 minutes **Number of Portions:** 4

Required Material for this Recipe:
- A cup of quinoa, after being washed and drained
- Vegetable stock, two pints
- One avocado, sliced
- Cherry tomatoes, one cup, cut in half
- Diced red onion, about one tiny
- 1/4 cups of finely chopped fresh cilantro
- One lime, only juice
- Olive oil, 2 tablespoons
- Pepper and salt

Step By Step Instructions for Recipe:
1. In a saucepan, bring the veggie stock and quinoa to a simmer.
2. Quinoa is done when it is soft and the cooking juice has been consumed, which takes about 15 minutes at a low boil.
3. Throw together some quinoa that's already been prepared, some sliced avocado, some cherry tomatoes, some red onion, and some minced cilantro.
4. In a separate dish, combine olive oil, citrus juice, salt, and pepper.
5. Toss the quinoa salad with the vinaigrette until everything is evenly coated.

6. Serve chilled with additional salt and pepper.

Nutritional Analysis: Quantity of Energy in Calories: 270, Quantity of Fat: 14g, Quantity of Carbs: 32g, Quantity of Fiber: 8g, Quantity of Protein: 7g

178. Broccoli and Turmeric Soup

Making and Duration Time: 13 minutes **Cooking Duration:** 25 minutes **Number of Portions:** 4

Required Material for this Recipe:
- Approximately one tablespoon of olive oil
- One small shallot, minced
- Two bulbs of chopped garlic
- An entire head of broccoli, diced; 1 teaspoon of powdered turmeric
- Four pints of stock made from vegetables
- Pepper and salt

Step By Step Instructions for Recipe:
1. Olive oil should be warmed over medium heat in a big saucepan.
2. Bake for another two to three minutes, or until the onion and garlic are soft.
3. Toss in the broccoli florets and roast for 5–7 minutes.
4. Blend in some powdered turmeric.
5. Soup can be made vegetarian by substituting veggie broth for water.
6. The cooking time for delicate broccoli is 15 to 20 minutes at a low boil.
7. Use a blender or an immersion blender to puree the broth until it is completely smooth.
8. Serve immediately with salt and pepper.

Nutritional Analysis: Quantity of Energy in Calories: 80, Quantity of Fat: 3g, Quantity of Carbs: 13g, Quantity of Fiber: 4g, Quantity of Protein: 4g

179. Chickpea and Vegetable Curry

Making and Duration Time: 10 minutes **Cooking Duration:** 30 minutes **Number of Portions:** 4

Required Material for this Recipe:
- 2 tablespoons of coconut oil
- One small shallot, minced, and one garlic

- One scarlet pepper, chopped
- Only one courgetti, sliced.
- One cup of diced sweet potato, 1 can of legumes (chickpeas), strained and washed
- Half a teaspoon of curry in powder
- Ground ginger, 1/2 teaspoon
- A pinch of pepper, hot chili
- Diced tomatoes, one can
- Pepper and salt

Step By Step Instructions for Recipe:
1. In a skillet, melt the coconut oil over low to medium heat.
2. Mix in the chopped shallot and garlic, then place in the oven for 2–3 minutes.
3. Cook for another 5–7 minutes, after adding the pepper, courgette, and potato, and all will be soft.
4. Mix chickpeas, powdered ginger, and chili pepper after the chickpeas have been washed and drained.
5. Put the chopped tomatoes and curry in a pot and heat until the tomatoes are boiling.
6. Wait 15–20 minutes in the oven for the sweet potato to soften and the aromas to combine. Season with salt and pepper, then serve over heated rice or flatbread.

Nutritional Analysis: Quantity of Energy in Calories: 240, Quantity of Fat: 7g, Quantity of Carbs: 38g, Quantity of Fiber: 11g, Quantity of Protein: 9g

180. Roasted Pumpkin Salad

Making and Duration Time: 15 minutes **Cooking Duration:** 30 minutes **Number of Portions:** 4

Required Material for this Recipe:
- Peel and dice one butternut squash.
- Approximately one tablespoon of olive oil
- Pepper and salt
- Four mugs, spinach
- Crumbled feta cheese equaling half a cup
- One-fourth cup of minced hazelnuts
- Balsamic vinegar, 2 tablespoons
- Two Tablespoons of honey

Step By Step Instructions for Recipe:
1. Turn the oven on to 400 degrees.
2. Put the butternut squash in a dish and add the olive oil, salt, and pepper.

3. Prepare a roasting tray with a single piece of butternut squash.
4. To get a tender and slightly browned butternut squash, bake it 25-30 minutes.
5. Dressing can be made by combining equal parts balsamic vinegar and honey.
6. In a separate dish, mix greens, baked butternut squash, feta cheese, and sliced hazelnuts. Add the balsamic vinegar to the lettuce and stir to incorporate. Serve.

Nutritional Analysis: Quantity of Energy in Calories: 230, Quantity of Fat: 16g, Quantity of Carbs: 19g, Quantity of Fiber: 4g, Quantity of Protein: 6g

181. Sweet Potato and Lentil Stew

Making and Duration Time: 17 minutes **Cooking Duration:** 30 minutes **Number of Portions:** 4

Required Material for this Recipe:
- Just one tablespoon of olive oil
- Diced onion
- Two garlic
- 2 cups of sliced sweet potato; 1 cup of dehydrated, washed legumes (lentils)
- 1 teaspoon powdered cumin, 4 mugs veggie stock
- Paprika, smoky, 1/2 tsp.
- Pepper and salt

Step By Step Instructions for Recipe:
1. Olive oil should be warmed over medium heat in a saucepan.
2. After 2 or 3 minutes, add the chopped onion and garlic and sauté until aromatic.
3. Cook the diced potato in a stir-fry for about 5–7 minutes or until fork-tender.
4. Add vegetable broth, legumes that have been washed and strained, powdered cumin, and smoky paprika to the saucepan. Get the broth boiling.
5. Simmer for 15–20 minutes until the lentils are tender and the aromas have blended at medium heat.
6. Served heated with toast or rice and some salt and pepper, of course.

Nutritional Analysis: Quantity of Energy in Calories: 220, Quantity of Fat: 4g, Quantity of Carbs: 35g, Quantity of Fiber: 13g, Quantity of Protein: 10g

182. Broccoli and Chickpea Stir-Fry

Making and Duration Time: 12 minutes **Cooking Duration:** 15 minutes **Number of Portions:** 4

Required Material for this Recipe:
- Oil from vegetables, 2 tablespoons
- Ginger, minced, 1 tablespoon
- Chopped garlic, two
- Broccoli that has been broken down into florets
- One scarlet bell pepper, cut
- Chickpeas, one can, rinsed and drained
- Soy sauce, 2 tablespoons
- Two tablespoons of honey
- A splash of rice vinegar
- Pepper and salt

Step By Step Instructions for Recipe:
1. Vegetable oil should be heated in a skillet over medium heat. Cook the garlic and ginger for 1–2 minutes, or until aromatic.
2. Broccoli stems and red bell pepper pieces can be cooked in a stir-fry for 5–7 min.
3. After the legumes have been drained and washed, add them to the pan and continue to stir-fry for another 2-3 minutes.
4. Create the condiment by combining soy sauce, honey, and rice vinegar.
5. Add the sauce to the sauté and toss to combine. Season with salt and pepper, then serve over heated rice or pasta.

Nutritional Analysis: Quantity of Energy in Calories: 230, Quantity of Fat: 9g, Quantity of Carbs: 30g, Quantity of Fiber: 7g, Quantity of Protein: 9g.

183. Cauliflower Fried Rice

Making and Duration Time: 13 minutes **Cooking Duration:** 16 minutes **Number of Portions:** 4

Required Material for this Recipe:
- One cauliflower stalk, sliced
- Oil from vegetables, 2 tablespoons
- One small shallot, minced
- 2 chopped garlic
- Two carrots, sliced
- Frozen peas, one cup

- Two eggs, beaten
- Add 3 tablespoons of soy sauce.
- 1 tablespoon of sesame oil
- Pepper and salt

Step By Step Instructions for Recipe:
1. Vegetable oil should be heated in a skillet over medium heat.
2. The aroma of the minced garlic and shallot can be enhanced by cooking them together for a few minutes.
3. Cook the thawed peas and diced carrots in a stir-fry for about 5 minutes, or until the vegetables are soft. Cook the cauliflower rice in a skillet for 3–5 minutes, or until it reaches the desired tenderness.
4. Separate the vegetables into one half of the pan and the eggs into the other.
5. Cook the eggs in a scrambler and then add them to the veggies.
6. To prepare the marinade, combine soy sauce and olive oil in a small dish.
7. Pour the marinade over the finished rice to coat it. Serve immediately.

Nutritional Analysis: Quantity of Energy in Calories: 170, Quantity of Fat: 11g, Quantity of Carbs: 14g, Quantity of Fiber: 5g, Quantity of Protein: 7g

184. Roasted Potato Salad

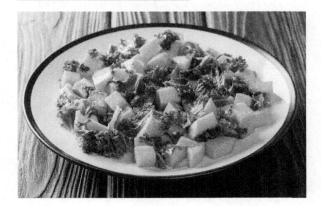

Making and Duration Time: 11 minutes **Cooking Duration:** 30 minutes **Number of Portions:** 4

Required Material for this Recipe:
- Two sweet potatoes, average in size, skinned and chopped
- Olive oil, 2 tablespoons
- Smoked paprika, one teaspoon

- Pepper and salt
- Four mugs, spinach
- Dried cranberries, half a cup
- One-fourth cup of minced nuts
- Feta cheese, shredded, about a quarter cup
- Balsamic vinegar, 2 tablespoons
- Two tablespoons of honey

Step By Step Instructions for Recipe:
1. Turn the oven on to 400 degrees.
2. Olive oil, smoky paprika, salt, and pepper should be added to the dish with the diced potatoes.
3. Bake the potatoes for 25 to 30 minutes, or until they are soft and golden brown, in a single layer on a baking pan.
4. Spinach, dried cranberries, minced walnuts, and shredded feta cheese should be mixed together.
5. To prepare the vinaigrette, combine equal parts balsamic vinegar and honey in a separate dish.
6. Toss the lettuce with the vinaigrette before adding the baked sweet potatoes. Serve.

Nutritional Analysis: Quantity of Energy in Calories: 250, Quantity of Fat: 12g, Quantity of Carbs: 33g, Quantity of Fiber: 4g, Quantity of Protein: 4g

185. Lentil and Vegetable Soup

Making and Duration Time: 10 minutes **Cooking Duration:** 30 minutes **Number of Portions:** 6

Required Material for this Recipe:
- Olive oil, 2 tablespoons
- An Onion, Minced
- Two carrots, chopped
- Minced celery from two stems, 2 chopped garlic
- A jar of tomato paste
- Vegetable broth, four glasses' worth
- Rinsed and strained legumes, equaling one cup
- Dried thyme, one teaspoon
- Pepper and salt
- Baby spinach, two quarts

Step By Step Instructions for Recipe:
1. Olive oil should be warmed in a skillet over low to medium heat.

2. Cook for 5–7 minutes, or until the onion, carrot, and celery have softened.
3. Toss in some minced garlic and cook for a few minutes until it begins to release its aroma.
4. Cooked legumes, dried thyme, and spices for seasoning, along with chopped tomatoes, in a saucepan on the stove.
5. The legumes should be tender after 20–25 minutes of simmering the broth at low heat.
6. Cook the spinach in the broth for two or three minutes with the salt and pepper until it wilts. Keep warm.

Nutritional Analysis: Quantity of Energy in Calories: 180, Quantity of Fat: 5g, Quantity of Carbs: 25g, Quantity of Fiber: 9g, Quantity of Protein: 9g

186. Grilled Veggie Skewers

Making and Duration Time: 15 minutes **Cooking Duration:** 11 minutes **Number of Portions:** 4

Required Material for this Recipe:
- 1 courgette, sliced lengthwise
- One round of golden squash
- One small red bell pepper, diced
- Cubes of one golden bell pepper
- A single red onion, diced
- Approximately one tablespoon of olive oil
- A pinch of rosemary, preserved
- Pepper and salt
- Four spears made of wood, submerged in water for half an hour

Step By Step Instructions for Recipe:
1. Prepare a medium fire on the griddle.
2. Add olive oil, dried oregano, salt, and pepper to a dish of chopped zucchini, yellow squash, red bell pepper, yellow bell pepper, and red onion.
3. Thread the different veggies onto the wet wooden skewers in alternating order.
4. Cook the veggie kebabs on the grill for 5 minutes per side until tender and lightly charred.
5. Serve them immediately.

Nutritional Analysis: Quantity of Energy in Calories: 70, Quantity of Fat: 4g, Quantity of Carbs: 9g, Quantity of Fiber: 4g, Quantity of Protein: 3g

187. Cucumber and Tomato Salad

Making and Duration Time: 11 minutes
Number of Portions: 4

Required Material for this Recipe:
- Tomatoes, sliced, 2 quarts
- 2 large, finely diced cucumbers
- Parsley, fresh, chopped: 1/4 cup
- Red onion, chopped, 1/4 cup
- Olive oil, 2 tablespoons
- The juice of half a lemon
- Pepper and salt

Step By Step Instructions for Recipe:
1. Throw some fresh parsley, red onion, cherry tomatoes, and sliced cucumbers.
2. The vinaigrette can be made in a separate dish by mixing olive oil, lemon juice, salt, and pepper.
3. Toss the cucumbers and tomatoes with the sauce and serve. Serve.

Nutritional Analysis: Quantity of Energy in Calories: 80, Quantity of Fat: 6g, Quantity of Carbs: 7g, Quantity of Fiber: 2g, Quantity of Protein: 2g

188. Chickpea and Spinach Stew

Making and Duration Time: 11 minutes
Cooking Duration: 30 minutes **Number of Portions:** 4

Required Material for this Recipe:
- Approximately one tablespoon of olive oil
- 1 medium-sized scallion, sliced
- Three bulbs of garlic, chopped
- Ground cumin, 1 teaspoon
- 1 teaspoon of cilantro powder
- Turmeric powder, 1/2 teaspoon
- 1/4 teaspoons of cinnamon powder
- An emptied and washed can of chickpeas
- A jar of tomato paste
- Vegetable broth, 2 pints
- Two and a half cups of baby spinach greens
- Pepper and salt
- Sliced lemons for garnishing

Step By Step Instructions for Recipe:
1. Olive oil should be warmed over medium heat in a saucepan. Once the onion is transparent, add the chopped onion and garlic and simmer for another 5 minutes.
2. Mix the powdered spices in the pot: cumin, coriander, ginger, and cinnamon.
3. Throw in some beans, some chopped tomatoes, and some veggie stock, and give it a good mix. Turn up the heat until the broth is boiling, and then turn it down.
4. For 20 minutes, or until the liquid has thickened slightly, boil the sauce.
5. Combine the spinach with fresh greens and stir. Allow the broth to cook for an additional 5 minutes to allow the greens to wilt.
6. Season with salt and pepper, then serve immediately with lemon wedges.

Nutritional Analysis: Quantity of Energy in Calories: 170, Quantity of Fat: 5g, Quantity of Carbs: 25g, Quantity of Fiber: 7g, Quantity of Protein: 7g

189. Zucchini Noodles and Tomato Sauce

Making and Duration Time: 13 minutes
Cooking Duration: 20 minutes **Number of Portions:** 4

Required Material for this Recipe:
- Noodles are made from four medium-sized zucchinis.
- Approximately one tablespoon of olive oil
- An onion, small enough to chop
- Three bulbs of garlic, chopped
- Crushed tomatoes in a can
- Dried basil, one teaspoon
- Oregano, powdered, one teaspoon
- Pepper and salt
- shredded Parmesan

Step By Step Instructions for Recipe:
1. Olive oil should be warmed over medium heat in a pan. Cook the onion and garlic for 5 minutes, or until the onion becomes transparent after being cubed.
2. Stir in the chopped tomatoes, salt, pepper, dried basil, and oregano. The sauce should be brought to a simmer before the heat is reduced.
3. Let the tomato mixture clarify a little by simmering it for 10 minutes.

4. Make zucchini noodles by spiralizing a zucchini while the tomato sauce cooks.
5. Put the zucchini noodles in a skillet and pour the tomato sauce over them, mixing well. Cook the zucchini noodles for 5–7 minutes, or until they reach the desired doneness.
6. Sprinkle with Parmesan cheese and serve immediately while still heated, season with salt and pepper.

Nutritional Analysis: Quantity of Energy in Calories: 90, Quantity of Fat: 4g, Quantity of Carbs: 12g, Quantity of Fiber: 4g, Quantity of Protein: 4g

190. Roasted Cauliflower Salad & Tahini Sauce

Making and Duration Time: 15 minutes **Cooking Duration:** 30 minutes **Number of Portions:** 4

Required Material for this Recipe:
For Salad:
- flowers from 1 big cauliflower head
- Olive oil, 2 tablespoons
- Pepper and salt
- Four servings of vegetable salad
- Approximately 6 cherry tomatoes, halved
- Cucumber, diced, 1/2 cup
- One-fourth cup of minced red onion
- Parsley, fresh, chopped; 1/4 cup
- Fresh Mint, Measured to Be 1/4 Cup

To make the tahini sauce:
- One-fourth cup tahini
- Two garlic bulbs, chopped
- Olive oil, 2 tablespoons
- Lemon juice, fresh (2 tbsp)
- 1/4 teaspoon of salt
- Water 1-quarter of a Cup

Step By Step Instructions for Recipe:
1. Turn the oven on to 400 degrees.
2. Olive oil, salt, and pepper should be added to the dish containing the minced cauliflower pieces before serving.
3. Bake the cauliflower for 25-30 minutes, or until soft and faintly colored, in a single layer on a baking pan.
4. While the cauliflower is cooking, prepare the tahini sauce by whisking together the tahini, lemon juice, olive oil, chopped

garlic, and salt. Slowly add water while whisking until sauce reaches desired consistency.
5. Toss together some leaves, cherry tomatoes, cucumber, red onion, parsley, and mint.
6. After the cauliflower has been cooked, toss it in with the salad leaves and other vegetables. The lettuce should be tossed with the tahini sauce after it has been drizzled over it. Serve

Nutritional Analysis: Quantity of Energy in Calories: 220, Quantity of Fat: 18g, Quantity of Carbs: 13g, Quantity of Fiber: 5g, Quantity of Protein: 6g

191. Sweet Potato and Black Bean Chili

Making and Duration Time: 11 minutes **Cooking Duration:** 30 minutes **Number of Portions:** 4

Required Material for this Recipe:
- Approximately one tablespoon of olive oil
- One big onion, chopped
- Three garlic bulbs, chopped
- Two sweet potatoes, average in size, skinned and diced
- Black beans from a can, washed and drained
- A jar of tomato paste
- Ground cumin, 1 teaspoon
- Pepper and salt
- Fresh cilantro, chopped, and avocado, diced (for serving).

Step By Step Instructions for Recipe:
1. Olive oil should be warmed over medium heat in a big saucepan. When the onion is transparent, about 5 minutes after adding the chopped onion and garlic, turn the heat down to low.
2. In a large saucepan, combine the sliced potatoes, canned black beans, canned cubed tomatoes, vegetable stock, chile powder, powdered cumin, salt, and pepper.
3. The chili should be brought to a simmer before the heat is reduced. The sweet potatoes need to be cooked for 20 minutes while the chili simmers.

4. Top the spicy stew with diced avocado and fresh parsley.

Nutritional Analysis: Quantity of Energy in Calories: 230, Quantity of Fat: 5g, Quantity of Carbs: 41g, Quantity of Fiber: 10g, Quantity of Protein: 9g

192. Grilled Eggplant in Chimichurri Sauce

Making and Duration Time: 10 minutes **Cooking Duration:** 11 minutes **Number of Portions:** 4

Required Material for this Recipe:
- Thin slices of two big eggplants (about 1/2 inch thick)
- Olive oil, 2 tablespoons
- Pepper and salt
- Two tablespoons of freshly chopped thyme
- Fresh coriander, chopped, 2 tablespoons
- Two garlic bulbs, chopped
- One-fourth cup of fresh cilantro, chopped
- Red wine vinegar, 2 tablespoons
- One-fourth cup of olive oil
- Pepper and salt

Step By Step Instructions for Recipe:
1. Prepare a medium fire in the griddle.
2. Sliced eggplant should be brushed with olive oil and then seasoned with salt and pepper.
3. Eggplant needs 3–4 minutes of cooking time per side to become faintly browned and tender.
4. Chimichurri dressing can be made while the eggplant is simmering. In a dish, combine the sliced herbs, red wine vinegar, olive oil, salt, and pepper.
5. Put the roasted eggplant on a plate and drizzle the chimichurri marinade over it.
6. Chimichurri dressing should be served on the side.

Nutritional Analysis: Quantity of Energy in Calories: 180, Quantity of Fat: 15g, Quantity of Carbs: 12g, Quantity of Fiber: 7g, Quantity of Protein: 3g

193. Quinoa Stuffed Bell Peppers

Making and Duration Time: 13 minutes **Cooking Duration:** 30 minutes **Number of Portions:** 4

Required Material for this Recipe:
- Four sliced and halved bell peppers
- Quinoa, one cup, strained and washed
- Two tablespoons of vegetable broth
- Black beans from a can, strained and washed
- A jar of tomato paste
- Add 1 tablespoon of chile pepper
- Ground cumin, 1 teaspoon
- Pepper and salt
- One-fourth cup of freshly cut parsley
- Thin pieces of avocado for a snack

Step By Step Instructions for Recipe:
1. Preheat the oven to 375 degrees.
2. In a pot, mix the rice with the veggie stock. To cook quinoa, first bring it to a simmer, then reduce the heat.
3. For about 15 to 20 minutes, or until the quinoa is soft and the liquid is consumed, the quinoa should be simmered.
4. In a dish, mix together the quinoa and black beans that have been prepared, along with the chopped tomatoes, chile powder, powdered cumin, salt, and pepper.
5. Bake the quinoa-stuffed bell pepper halves according to the manufacturer's instructions.
6. To ensure the peppers are soft and the mixture is hot throughout, cook them for 20–25 minutes.
7. Serve the filled bell peppers steaming, garnished with diced avocado and fresh parsley.

Nutritional Analysis: Quantity of Energy in Calories: 290, Quantity of Fat: 4g, Quantity of Carbs: 53g, Quantity of Fiber: 15g, Quantity of Protein: 14g

194. **Spinach and Chickpea Curry**

Making and Duration Time: 13 minutes **Cooking Duration:** 21 minutes **Number of Portions:** 4

Required Material for this Recipe:
- Approximately one tablespoon of olive oil
- An Onion, Minced
- Two garlic bulbs, chopped
- Fresh ginger, minced, 1 tablespoon
- Ground cumin, 2 teaspoons
- One teaspoon of cilantro powder
- Turmeric, 1/2 teaspoon
- A pinch of red pepper flakes
- An emptied and washed can of chickpeas
- A jar of tomato paste
- One-half cup of vegetable broth
- Pepper and salt
- About 6 cups of raw greens.
- One-fourth cup of fresh cilantro, chopped

Step By Step Instructions for Recipe:
1. The sliced onion only needs 5 minutes in a skillet with warm olive oil over medium heat to mellow.
2. Combine the powdered cumin, coriander, turmeric, and chili pepper with the chopped garlic and sliced ginger.
3. Toss in some canned beans, tomato chunks, vegetable broth, salt, and pepper. Prepare in ten minutes.
4. After 2 or 3 minutes of tossing, the raw spinach will have wilted.
5. Serve over brown rice and sprinkle with chopped cilantro.

Nutritional Analysis: Quantity of Energy in Calories: 220, Quantity of Fat: 5g, Quantity of Carbs: 36g, Quantity of Fiber: 10g, Quantity of Protein: 11g

195. **Broccoli and Sweet Potato Soup**

Making and Duration Time: 13 minutes **Cooking Duration:** 30 minutes **Number of Portions:** 4

Required Material for this Recipe:
- Olive oil, 2 tablespoons
- One small onion minced; two garlic bulbs minced
- A sizable, sweet potato, skinned and diced.
- One broccoli head's worth of chopping, four gallons of vegetable broth
- Pepper and salt
- Fresh parsley, chopped, about a quarter cup

Step By Step Instructions for Recipe:
1. Olive oil should be warmed in a saucepan over medium heat. The diced onion needs 5 minutes of cooking time to mellow.
2. Stir in the broccoli, garlic, and sweet potato.
3. Bring vegetable broth to a simmer and add it. Reduce heat and boil for 20–25 minutes, or until veggies are soft.
4. The broth can be blended into a creamy consistency using an immersion mixer. Put in some pepper and salt.
5. Serve to steam, topped with minced fresh parsley.

Nutritional Analysis: Quantity of Energy in Calories: 160, Quantity of Fat: 7g, Quantity of Carbs: 23g, Quantity of Fiber: 5g, Quantity of Protein: 4g

196. **Quinoa and Black Bean Salad**

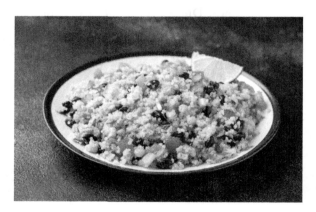

Making and Duration Time: 15 minutes **Cooking Duration:** 15 minutes **Number of Portions:** 4

Required Material for this Recipe:
- A cup of quinoa, after being cleaned and drained
- Black beans from a can, strained and washed
- One scarlet pepper, chopped
- An onion, red, minced, half

- One jalapeno pepper, seeded and chopped
- One-fourth cup of fresh cilantro, chopped
- Olive oil, 2 tablespoons
- Lime juice, fresh (2 tbsp)
- Cumin seed, pulverized, 1/2 teaspoon
- Pepper and salt

Step By Step Instructions for Recipe:
1. Follow the package directions for cooking the quinoa. Set it aside to settle down.
2. Combine a bowl's worth of minced cilantro, jalapeno, red onion, red bell pepper, and jalapeno pepper with some cooked quinoa.
3. Olive oil, lime juice, powdered cumin, salt, and pepper should be mixed in a separate dish. Add the liquid to the quinoa and stir to incorporate.
4. Cold or room temperature serving is recommended.

Nutritional Analysis: Quantity of Energy in Calories: 280, Quantity of Fat: 9g, Quantity of Carbs: 38g, Quantity of Fiber: 9g, Quantity of Protein: 11g

197. Roasted Vegetable and Lentil Salad

Making and Duration Time: 14 minutes **Cooking Duration:** 25 minutes **Number of Portions:** 4

Required Material for this Recipe:
- Minced assorted vegetables, two tablespoons' worth (such as zucchini, eggplant, bell pepper, and red onion)
- Olive oil, 2 tablespoons
- Pepper and salt
- Lentils, prepared to a cup's worth
- Feta cheese, shredded, about a quarter cup
- Finely chopped fresh cilantro, 2 tablespoons
- Balsamic vinegar, about a tablespoon
- TWO TABLESPOONS of honey
- Garlic that has been chopped

Step By Step Instructions for Recipe:
1. Turn the oven on to 400 degrees.
2. Add some olive oil, salt, and pepper to the diced vegetables and mix well. Cook for 20–25 minutes at 400°F until soft and caramelized.

3. In a dish, mix the legumes, the sautéed veggies, the feta cheese, and the fresh parsley that has been minced.
4. In a separate dish, mix the balsamic vinegar, honey, chopped garlic, salt, and pepper. Toss with the lettuce and serve with the toppings.

Nutritional Analysis: Quantity of Energy in Calories: 210, Quantity of Fat: 8g, Quantity of Carbs: 27g, Quantity of Fiber: 8g, Quantity of Protein: 10g

198. Roasted Carrot and Quinoa Salad

Making and Duration Time: 15 minutes **Cooking Duration:** 25 minutes **Number of Portions:** 4

Required Material for this Recipe:
- Four big carrots, cleaned and cut
- Olive oil, 2 tablespoons
- Pepper and salt
- Quinoa, one cup, strained and washed
- The equivalent of two glasses of water
- Fresh parsley, chopped, equaling a half cup
- One-half cup of fresh mint, chopped
- One-fourth cup of roasted almonds, chopped
- Feta cheese, shredded, about a quarter cup
- Lemon juice, 2 tablespoons
- TWO TABLESPOONS of honey
- 1 tsp. of spicy Dijon mustard

Step By Step Instructions for Recipe:
1. Pre-heat oven to 400 degrees Fahrenheit. Toss sliced carrots with olive oil, salt, and pepper, then spread them out on a baking sheet. Roast for 20 to 25 minutes, or until browned and tender.
2. Bring two cups of water to a boil in a saucepan, then add quinoa. Reduce heat, cover, and simmer for 15 to 20 minutes, or until water is absorbed and quinoa is cooked.

Nutritional Analysis: Quantity of Energy in Calories: 310, Quantity of Fat: 14g, Quantity of Carbs: 38g, Quantity of Fiber: 7g, Quantity of Protein: 9g

CHAPTER 11: 28-DAY MEAL PLAN

Here is a sample 28-day meal plan for an anti-inflammatory diet:

WEEK 1

Day 1
- **Breakfast:** Oatmeal with blueberries and almond milk
- **Snack:** Apple slices with almond butter
- **Lunch:** Salad with mixed greens, cherry tomatoes, cucumber, avocado, and grilled chicken
- **Snack:** Carrots and hummus
- **Dinner:** Grilled salmon with roasted sweet potatoes and green beans

Day 2
- **Breakfast:** Greek yogurt with strawberries and walnuts
- **Snack:** Banana with almond butter
- **Lunch:** Quinoa and black bean salad
- **Snack:** Celery and peanut butter
- **Dinner:** Baked chicken with roasted Brussels sprouts and brown rice

Day 3
- **Breakfast:** Smoothie with spinach, banana, almond milk, and chia seeds
- **Snack:** Handful of almonds
- **Lunch:** Turkey and vegetable stir-fry with brown rice
- **Snack:** Berries with whipped coconut cream
- **Dinner:** Grilled shrimp with roasted asparagus and quinoa

Day 4
- **Breakfast:** Egg omelet with mixed vegetables and avocado
- **Snack:** Orange slices with walnuts
- **Lunch:** Tuna salad with mixed greens, cherry tomatoes, cucumber, and olive oil dressing
- **Snack:** Pear with almond butter
- **Dinner:** Baked salmon with roasted broccoli and sweet potato

Day 5
- **Breakfast:** Overnight oats with mixed berries and almond milk
- **Snack:** Raw veggies with hummus
- **Lunch:** Lentil soup with a mixed green salad
- **Snack:** Apple slices with almond butter
- **Dinner:** Grilled chicken with roasted carrots and brown rice

Day 6
- **Breakfast:** Smoothie with kale, banana, almond milk, and hemp seeds
- **Snack:** Carrots with hummus
- **Lunch:** Grilled vegetable wrap with mixed greens and avocado
- **Snack:** Greek yogurt with mixed berries
- **Dinner:** Baked cod with roasted vegetables and quinoa

Day 7
- **Breakfast:** Egg muffin with mixed vegetables and feta cheese
- **Snack:** Handful of cashews
- **Lunch:** Grilled chicken with mixed greens, cherry tomatoes, cucumber, and olive oil dressing
- **Snack:** Berries with whipped coconut cream
- **Dinner:** Baked sweet potato with black bean chili and mixed vegetables

WEEK 2:

Day 8
- **Breakfast:** Oatmeal with banana and almond milk
- **Snack:** Apple slices with almond butter
- **Lunch:** Chicken and vegetable stir-fry with brown rice
- **Snack:** Carrots and hummus
- **Dinner:** Grilled salmon with roasted sweet potatoes and green beans

Day 9
- **Breakfast:** Greek yogurt with mixed berries and walnuts
- **Snack:** Banana with almond butter
- **Lunch:** Quinoa and black bean salad
- **Snack:** Celery and peanut butter
- **Dinner:** Baked chicken with roasted Brussels sprouts and brown rice

Day 10
- **Breakfast:** Smoothie with spinach, mixed berries, almond milk, and chia seeds
- **Snack:** Handful of almonds
- **Lunch:** Turkey and vegetable wrap with mixed greens and avocado
- **Snack:** Berries with whipped coconut cream
- **Dinner:** Grilled shrimp with roasted asparagus and quinoa

Day 11
- **Breakfast:** Egg omelet with mixed vegetables and avocado
- **Snack:** Orange slices with walnuts
- **Lunch:** Tuna salad with mixed greens, cherry tomatoes, cucumber, and olive oil dressing
- **Snack:** Pear with almond butter
- **Dinner:** Baked salmon with roasted broccoli and sweet potato

Day 12
- **Breakfast:** Overnight oats with mixed berries and almond milk
- **Snack:** Raw veggies with hummus
- **Lunch:** Lentil soup with a mixed green salad
- **Snack:** Apple slices with almond butter
- **Dinner:** Grilled chicken with roasted carrots and brown rice

Day 13
- **Breakfast:** Smoothie with kale, banana, almond milk, and hemp seeds
- **Snack:** Carrots with hummus
- **Lunch:** Grilled vegetable wrap with mixed greens and avocado
- **Snack:** Greek yogurt with mixed berries
- **Dinner:** Baked cod with roasted vegetables and quinoa

Day 14
- **Breakfast:** Egg muffin with mixed vegetables and feta cheese
- **Snack:** Handful of cashews
- **Lunch:** Grilled chicken with mixed greens, cherry tomatoes, cucumber, and olive oil dressing
- **Snack:** Berries with whipped coconut cream
- **Dinner:** Baked sweet potato with black bean chili and mixed vegetables

WEEK 3:

Day 15
- **Breakfast:** Oatmeal with blueberries and almond milk
- **Snack:** Apple slices with almond butter
- **Lunch:** Salad with mixed greens, cherry tomatoes, cucumber, avocado, and grilled chicken
- **Snack:** Carrots and hummus
- **Dinner:** Grilled salmon with roasted sweet potatoes and green beans

Day 16
- **Breakfast:** Greek yogurt with strawberries and walnuts
- **Snack:** Banana with almond butter
- **Lunch:** Quinoa and black bean salad
- **Snack:** Celery and peanut butter
- **Dinner:** Baked chicken with roasted Brussels sprouts and brown rice

Day 17
- **Breakfast:** Smoothie with spinach, banana, almond milk, and chia seeds
- **Snack:** Handful of almonds
- **Lunch:** Turkey and vegetable stir-fry with brown rice
- **Snack:** Berries with whipped coconut cream
- **Dinner:** Grilled shrimp with roasted asparagus and quinoa

Day 18
- **Breakfast:** Egg omelet with mixed vegetables and avocado
- **Snack:** Orange slices with walnuts
- **Lunch:** Tuna salad with mixed greens, cherry tomatoes, cucumber, and olive oil dressing
- **Snack:** Pear with almond butter
- **Dinner:** Baked salmon with roasted broccoli and sweet potato

Day 19
- **Breakfast:** Overnight oats with mixed berries and almond milk
- **Snack:** Raw veggies with hummus
- **Lunch:** Lentil soup with a mixed green salad
- **Snack:** Apple slices with almond butter
- **Dinner:** Grilled chicken with roasted carrots and brown rice

Day 20
- **Breakfast:** Smoothie with kale, banana, almond milk, and hemp seeds
- **Snack:** Carrots with hummus
- **Lunch:** Grilled vegetable wrap with mixed greens and avocado
- **Snack:** Greek yogurt with mixed berries
- **Dinner:** Baked cod with roasted vegetables and quinoa

Day 21
- **Breakfast:** Egg muffin with mixed vegetables and feta cheese
- **Snack:** Handful of cashews
- **Lunch:** Grilled chicken with mixed greens, cherry tomatoes, cucumber, and olive oil dressing
- **Snack:** Berries with whipped coconut cream
- **Dinner:** Baked sweet potato with black bean chili and mixed vegetables

WEEK 4:

Day 22

- **Breakfast:** Oatmeal with blueberries and almond milk
- **Snack:** Apple slices with almond butter
- **Lunch:** Salad with mixed greens, cherry tomatoes, cucumber, avocado, and grilled chicken
- **Snack:** Carrots and hummus
- **Dinner:** Grilled salmon with roasted sweet potatoes and green beans

Day 23

- **Breakfast:** Greek yogurt with strawberries and walnuts
- **Snack:** Banana with almond
- **Lunch:** Vegetable stir-fry with quinoa
- **Snack:** Mixed berries with whipped coconut cream
- **Dinner:** Baked chicken with roasted Brussels sprouts and brown rice

Day 24

- **Breakfast:** Smoothie with spinach, banana, almond milk, and chia seeds
- **Snack:** Handful of almonds
- **Lunch:** Tuna salad with mixed greens, cherry tomatoes, cucumber, and olive oil dressing
- **Snack:** Pear with almond butter
- **Dinner:** Grilled shrimp with roasted asparagus and quinoa

Day 25

- **Breakfast:** Egg omelet with mixed vegetables and avocado
- **Snack:** Orange slices with walnuts
- **Lunch:** Lentil soup with a mixed green salad
- **Snack:** Raw veggies with hummus
- **Dinner:** Baked salmon with roasted broccoli and sweet potato

Day 26

- **Breakfast:** Overnight oats with mixed berries and almond milk
- **Snack:** Carrots with hummus
- **Lunch:** Grilled vegetable wrap with mixed greens and avocado
- **Snack:** Greek yogurt with mixed berries
- **Dinner:** Baked cod with roasted vegetables and quinoa

Day 27

- **Breakfast:** Smoothie with kale, banana, almond milk, and hemp seeds
- **Snack:** Raw veggies with hummus
- **Lunch:** Grilled chicken with mixed greens, cherry tomatoes, cucumber, and olive oil dressing
- **Snack:** Berries with whipped coconut cream
- **Dinner:** Baked sweet potato with black bean chili and mixed vegetables

Day 28

- **Breakfast:** Egg muffin with mixed vegetables and feta cheese
- **Snack:** Handful of cashews
- **Lunch:** Salad with mixed greens, cherry tomatoes, cucumber, avocado, and grilled chicken
- **Snack:** Carrots and hummus
- **Dinner:** Grilled salmon with roasted sweet potatoes and green beans

Note: This meal plan is for general informational purposes only and is not intended to be medical advice. Please consult with a healthcare professional before changing your diet or lifestyle.

CHAPTER 12: PHYSICAL EXERCISE TO GET FIT

Incorporating physical exercise into your routine can complement an anti-inflammatory diet and promote overall health and fitness. Here are some examples of exercises that can help you get fit while on the anti-inflammatory diet, along with safety measures and tips for maximizing their benefits:

1. Aerobic Exercise: Jogging, cycling, swimming, and brisk walking can improve cardiovascular health and boost endurance. Aim for 30 minutes of moderate to vigorous aerobic exercise most days of the week.

Safety Measures: Always warm up before starting your aerobic workout and gradually increase the intensity. Wear appropriate shoes and clothing to avoid injury and stay hydrated throughout your workout. If you have any underlying medical conditions, such as heart disease or arthritis, talk to your doctor before starting any new exercise routine.

Maximizing Benefits: Vary your aerobic activities to prevent boredom and target different muscle groups. For example, alternate between jogging and cycling, or switch up your swimming strokes. Consider adding high-intensity intervals to your workout to increase your heart rate and challenge your cardiovascular system.

2. Strength Training: Resistance exercises like weightlifting or bodyweight exercises like push-ups and squats can increase muscle mass and bone density while improving balance and coordination. Aim for 2-3 sessions per week, targeting all major muscle groups.

Safety Measures: Start with lighter weights or resistance bands and focus on proper form and technique before gradually increasing the weight or resistance. Use a spotter or trainer for heavier lifts to prevent injury. Make sure to rest and recover between strength training sessions to avoid overuse injuries.

Maximizing Benefits: Focus on compound exercises that target multiple muscle groups, such as squats or lunges, to maximize your workout efficiency. Consider adding plyometric exercises, such as jump squats or burpees, to increase the intensity and challenge your muscles.

3. Yoga: This ancient practice combines physical postures with breathwork and meditation to promote flexibility, strength, and relaxation. Yoga has been shown to reduce inflammation and improve overall well-being.

Safety Measures: Listen to your body and don't push yourself beyond your limits. Work with a qualified instructor who can guide you through proper alignment and modifications for any injuries or limitations. Avoid certain poses, such as inversions, if you have certain medical conditions, such as high blood pressure.

Maximizing Benefits: Focus on your breath and try to quiet your mind during your yoga practice to promote relaxation and stress reduction. Consider incorporating props like blocks or straps to deepen your stretches and challenge your balance.

4. High-Intensity Interval Training (HIIT): These workouts involve short, intense bursts of activity followed by brief rest or recovery periods. HIIT has been shown to improve cardiovascular health, increase muscle strength and endurance, and promote fat loss.

Safety Measures: Warm up thoroughly before starting your HIIT workout and gradually increase the intensity. Use proper form and technique to avoid injury. Make sure to rest and recover between HIIT sessions to avoid overuse injuries.

Maximizing Benefits: Alternate between different exercises, such as jumping jacks and burpees, to challenge different muscle groups and keep your workout interesting. Consider using a heart rate monitor to track your intensity and challenge yourself to reach higher intensity levels during each workout.

5. Low-Impact Exercise: Low-impact exercises, such as swimming, cycling, or walking, can be easier on the joints and are ideal for individuals with joint pain or inflammation. These activities still provide a great cardiovascular workout while reducing the risk of injury.

Safety Measures: Warm up before starting your low-impact exercise and gradually increase the intensity. Wear appropriate shoes and clothing to avoid injury and stay hydrated throughout your workout. If you have any underlying medical conditions, such as arthritis, talk to your doctor before starting any new exercise routine.

Maximizing Benefits: Consider incorporating resistance bands or light weights into your low-impact exercise routine to increase the challenge and build muscle strength. Experiment with different types of low-impact exercises, such as water aerobics or yoga, to keep your routine interesting and target different muscle groups.

Overall, choosing exercises you enjoy and can commit to regularly is important. Always prioritize safety and listen to your body, modifying to avoid injury or discomfort. Incorporating regular physical activity into your routine can enhance the benefits of an anti-inflammatory diet and promote overall health and wellness.

CONCLUSION

As we conclude this book about the anti-inflammatory diet, it is important to reflect on the key takeaways and the implications for our overall health and well-being.

First and foremost, we have learned that inflammation is a natural and necessary process in the body. Still, it can lead to various health problems when it becomes chronic and widespread. By adopting an anti-inflammatory diet, we can help to reduce chronic inflammation and promote better health outcomes.

The anti-inflammatory diet emphasizes whole, nutrient-dense foods, such as fruits, veggies, whole grains, lean protein sources, and healthy fats. These foods are rich in vitamins, minerals, and antioxidants, which can help to reduce inflammation and support overall health.

In contrast, the standard Western diet, high in processed foods, sugar, and unhealthy fats, has been linked to increased inflammation and a higher risk of chronic diseases, such as heart disease, diabetes, and cancer.

By making simple changes to our diet, such as reducing our intake of processed foods and sugar, increasing our intake of fruits and vegetables, and choosing healthier fats, we can help to reduce inflammation and promote better health.

But the anti-inflammatory diet is not just about what we eat. It also emphasizes the importance of other lifestyle factors, such as exercise, stress management, and sleep, which can also impact inflammation and overall health.

Regular exercise has been shown to reduce inflammation, while chronic stress and poor sleep can increase inflammation. By incorporating regular exercise into our routine and practicing stress management techniques, such as meditation and yoga, we can further support the anti-inflammatory benefits of our diet.

Overall, the anti-inflammatory diet is not a fad or a quick fix but a sustainable and holistic approach to promoting better health and reducing the risk of chronic diseases. By adopting this way of eating and living, we can support our bodies in functioning optimally and promote long-term health and vitality.

As we close this book, I encourage you to apply what you have learned to your life. Experiment with new recipes, try new foods and find what works best for you. And above all, remember that small changes can make a big difference in promoting better health and reducing inflammation. Thank you for joining me on this journey toward better health and well-being.

Printed in Great Britain
by Amazon

24893256R00057